KETOGENIC
PRESSURE COOKER

KETOGENIC
PRESSURE COOKER

150 QUICK AND EASY RECIPES FOR DELICIOUS,
NUTRIENT-PACKED LOW-CARB MEALS

AILEEN ABLOG

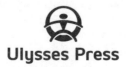

Ulysses Press

Published in the United States by
ULYSSES PRESS
P.O. Box 3440
Berkeley, CA 94703
www.ulyssespress.com

ISBN: 978-1-61243-680-7
Library of Congress Control Number: 2016957520

Printed in the United States by United Graphics Inc.
10 9 8 7 6 5 4 3 2 1

Acquisitions editor: Bridget Thoreson
Managing editor: Claire Chun
Project editor: Caety Klingman
Editor: Lauren Harrison
Proofreader: Renee Rutledge
Production: Caety Klingman
Front cover design: Michelle Thompson
Cover photograph: © AS Food Studio/shutterstock.com

Distributed by Publishers Group West

NOTE TO READERS: This book has been written and published strictly for informational and educational purposes only. It is not intended to serve as medical advice or to be any form of medical treatment. You should always consult your physician before altering or changing any aspect of your medical treatment and/or undertaking a diet regimen, including the guidelines as described in this book. Do not stop or change any prescription medications without the guidance and advice of your physician. Any use of the information in this book is made on the reader's good judgment after consulting with his or her physician and is the reader's sole responsibility. This book is not intended to diagnose or treat any medical condition and is not a substitute for a physician.

This book is independently authored and published and no sponsorship or endorsement of this book by, and no affiliation with, any trademarked brands or other products mentioned within is claimed or suggested. All trademarks that appear in ingredient lists and elsewhere in this book belong to their respective owners and are used here for informational purposes only. The author and publisher encourage readers to patronize the quality brands mentioned and pictured in this book.

This book is dedicated to everyone looking to make a change,
or in the process of change, for better health.
I applaud and congratulate you on your journey.

Contents

CHAPTER 5
Poultry. **64**

Introduction

I've been overweight for the majority of my life, and I know the roller coaster of dieting all too well: Working hard, eating "right," and yet always staying hungry. When I first heard of the ketogenic diet, I thought it was a crazy fad and didn't think twice about it. It wasn't until almost a year later, when I stumbled upon it again and heard of people who followed it not only losing weight but reversing ailments such as type 2 diabetes and high-blood pressure, that I was tempted to give it a try.

It sounded too good to be true, and the basis of the diet was contrary to everything I was taught.

But I was overweight, borderline obese, and I knew I had to make a change or I was headed for a lifetime of medications to keep my blood pressure, blood sugars, and fats in check. Coupled with a family history of coronary disease and hypertension, the cards were stacked against me.

I did some further research, and the science behind it was sound. I told myself I would give it an honest try for three months, and then I'd reevaluate. I still had doubts, so I had blood tests done along the way and knew if there was any contrary indication, I would discontinue the diet.

That decision was almost two years ago, and I haven't looked back. My blood work is normal—in fact, it's great. I've lost close to 45 pounds on a 5'3" frame and feel better than ever. I don't need to lose any more weight, but I've decided to maintain a ketogenic way of eating because I like the way I feel.

Before starting the ketogenic diet, I had the great fortune of picking up an electric pressure cooker. Since then, I have had many tasty successes and my cooking style has changed somewhat. I'm happy that pressure cooking has made preparing foods for the ketogenic diet faster and easier, and I hope that you find the same too!

Note: I strongly suggest you consult a medical professional who is familiar with the diet and its risks, along with your medical history, to see if this diet is suitable for you.

CHAPTER 1
The Ketogenic Diet

The ketogenic diet is an ultra-low carb, moderate-protein, and high-fat way of eating. In essence, it is restricting carbohydrate intake (sugars, starches, etc.) and increasing healthy fats. This process causes the body to go into the metabolic state of ketosis, where the liver converts these fatty acids into ketones (beta hydroxybutyrate and acetoacetate) that the body uses for energy. It should not be confused with diabetic ketoacidosis, which is a dangerous complication of diabetes.

Low-Carb versus Ketogenic

General "low-carb" eating plans, or reducing daily carbohydrate intake to 150 to 100 grams, should not be confused with a ketogenic diet. While a low-carbohydrate diet reduces the amount of carbs a person consumes, it may not necessarily cause the ketosis state. A ketogenic diet is considered ultra-low carb, where intake is restricted to fewer than 50 grams of net carbs (total carbs minus fiber) daily; 20 to 25 grams of net carbs is ideal, along with moderate protein (usually about 0.8 to 1.0 gram of protein per pound of lean body mass) and high fat. A typical ketogenic diet contains 75% of calories from fat, 20% of calories from protein, and about 5% of calories from carbs.

Once the body has adapted to a ketogenic diet, depending on the individual, some people can increase their carb intake and still remain in the ketosis state.

Benefits of the Ketogenic Diet

People who have had success on a ketogenic diet have found some or all of these benefits, depending on the individual:

Muscle sparing: Some other diets cause some people to experience muscle loss when cutting back caloric intake. This is not the case with the keto diet.

Mental clarity, focus, and mood stabilization: The diet stabilizes mood swings without the carbohydrate/sugar highs and lows, in addition to increasing the brain's ability to utilize ketones for energy rather than relying solely on glucose.

Burning fat stores: By eating at a caloric deficit and utilizing fat as an energy source, the body is able to use available fat stores, reducing body fat over time.

Blood sugar reduction: When carbohydrates are restricted, blood glucose and liver glycogen (chains of glucose) stores are used up, reducing blood sugar levels.

Insulin reduction: In the presence of carbohydrates, the body responds by releasing the hormone insulin to control the absorption of glucose into the cells from the bloodstream. Without carbohydrates, there is no or very little insulin response. This can also be of particular interest for those who have become insulin resistant, meaning their body doesn't respond to insulin. Giving the body a break from insulin may increase insulin sensitivity for this group.

Satisfaction: By using fats as the primary fuel source, and because fats are nutrient-dense (1 gram of fat has 9 calories), many people on a ketogenic diet feel satisfied, unlike the case with other diets that leave an unfulfilled feeling or a constant hunger.

It doesn't feel like a diet: It doesn't feel like one is on a diet at all when they are able to eat richer, higher-fat, more flavorful foods than on other diets.

How to Get Started with a Ketogenic Diet

There are different approaches to implementing a ketogenic diet, and there may be one that works better for you.

Macro counting/weighing/tracking: There are numerous online ketogenic macro calculators that can help you determine your particular macronutrient profile (the number of fats, carbs, and proteins you should be consuming in a day) based on your height, weight, age, body fat percentage, lifestyle, and weight-loss goal (if any).

"Lazy Keto": This approach to the diet doesn't involve tracking or weighing. Essentially, eat when you're truly hungry, stop when you're satisfied, and don't eat the foods on the Foods to Avoid list (page 6).

For both approaches, familiarize yourself with nutritional facts, ingredient labels, and which foods are acceptable on the diet.

The following lists are by no means complete; they're just to give you an idea and a place to start. When in doubt, read the nutritional information on the product label or look up the information online on any of the databases available, such as the USDA Food Composition Database.

ACCEPTED FOODS

Dairy: heavy cream, full-fat cheeses, butter, ghee, full-fat sour cream

Fats: coconut oil, avocado oil, olive oil, butter, lard, medium-chain triglycerides (MCT)

Fruit: avocado

Proteins: beef, eggs, fish, lamb, pork, poultry, shellfish

Vegetables: asparagus, bok choy, broccoli, cabbage, cauliflower, kale, spinach, zucchini

FOODS TO AVOID

Fruits: fruits contain carbs and sugars

All low-fat foods: to make foods low in fat, sugars are added for flavor; plus, on a ketogenic diet fat is fuel

All processed foods: many processed foods have hidden sugars to boost flavor and starches to improve texture

Premade sauces, dressings, and condiments: many of these have added sugars for flavor and starches for thickeners; when in doubt, check the label

Starches: cereals, breads, beans, pasta, rice, grains, potatoes

Sugars: the body identifies sugars and processes them all the same; this includes high-fructose corn syrup, honey, maple syrup, and agave

Sugary drinks: soda, fruit juice

FOODS TO ENJOY IN MODERATION

All berries: these are high in fiber

Chocolate: the darker the better

Nuts: not all nuts are equal—some are higher in carbs than others

A note about alcohol: Wine, beer, and mixed drinks have varying amounts of carbohydrates. Dry wines and dark beer usually contain fewer carbs. Hard, unsweetened liquors such as whiskey, vodka, brandy, gin, rum, etc., don't contain carbs and usually won't knock the body out of ketosis, but ketone processing will be delayed.

Increase Your Intake

Along with eating more accepted foods and none of the foods that should be avoided, on a ketogenic diet you'll need to increase the following:

Fat intake: On keto, fats are essential to fuel the body. Coconut and palm kernel oils in particular are sources of medium-chain triglycerides, or MCT oils. These medium-chain triglycerides—fatty acids C6 caproic acid, C8 caprylic acid, and C10 capric acid—are of particular interest as they are converted to ketones readily. Other fats such as lard, ghee, and butter are good too.

Water intake: For every 1 gram of glycogen (chains of glucose) there are 3 to 4 grams of water associated with it, and when the glycogen stores are used up, the water goes too. You'll need to keep hydrated, and water is best.

Electrolyte intake: As the body loses water, sodium goes along with it, and to keep things in balance, potassium is lost. You'll need to make sure to keep up electrolytes by drinking bone broth or pickle juice, or simply adding some salt to your drinking water. Don't be afraid to add salt to your food too. A magnesium supplement is helpful as well.

Monitoring Your Progress

Have some goals in mind and give yourself a time frame to achieve them. Then, check in once a week to monitor your progress. Here are some ways you can evaluate how far you've come:

Scale: This is the usual method to track weight loss, but use it in conjunction with other methods.

Body fat percentage: You can use calipers to calculate body fat, but there are also some scales that have this built in. You can also get a DEXA body scan, which is more accurate but pricey.

If you know ahead of time where you'll be eating out, see if the restaurant has their menu along with nutritional information posted on their website. Then you can plan what to order and save time at the restaurant. If not, look through the menu for low-carb items—with the growing popularity of low-carb and ketogenic diets, many restaurants have dishes that cater to these needs. If you don't see anything, look for items with simple sauces. Inquire with the server if the sauces have been thickened with flour or starches, or if there are any sugars in them. Even something as simple as a green salad with a grilled protein and a vinaigrette works well for the ketogenic diet.

As you become more familiar and confident with the eating plan, you'll easily find items that are suitable.

Measurements: When the scale may seem like it's stuck, compare measurements. Take measurements of your hips, waist, chest, thighs, calves, upper arms, and forearms and see how these change over time.

Pictures: It can be difficult to see progress day to day, but by having progress pictures, you can see and compare side by side, which will give you a better idea of how your body is changing.

Blood tests: Blood glucose, A1C, LDL, HDL, triglycerides, sodium, and potassium are blood tests of general interest.

Mental and physical reflection: How are you feeling? How are your clothes fitting? Do you notice other changes?

Dealing with the "Keto Flu"

Some people experience headache, fatigue, sluggishness, weakness, and/or thirst within the first few days on the ketogenic diet. Sometimes this lasts a couple of weeks while your body becomes adapted. Most of the time it's due to an electrolyte imbalance as the body adjusts. It's easily remedied within minutes by taking in some salt, drinking stock, eating pickles, etc.

Cooking Keto for Non-Keto Diners

Many ketogenic dieters find themselves in households preparing foods where other family members aren't ketogenic. I've tried to make the recipes in this book appeal to a wide audience while keeping them as keto-friendly as possible. Appeasing non-keto eaters may be as simple as having a side dish consisting of rice or some higher-carb vegetables such as potatoes, beans, or corn, and reducing portion sizes.

A word of caution: If non-keto family members/diners have dietary restrictions in regard to fat and salt, and/or have a high carbohydrate intake, they should perhaps avoid ketogenic dishes, as these foods tend to be higher in fat, calories, and sodium.

CHAPTER 2

An Introduction to Pressure Cooking

Pressure cooking has come into vogue in the last few years. Whether it's because of the newer, safer, multifunction electric pressure cooking models available in the marketplace or wanting to go back to basics and cook from scratch without spending hours in the kitchen, there is no denying that pressure cooking is faster than conventional methods and quite flavorful. Using the pressure cooker also makes things so easy. I enjoy cooking frozen chicken breasts after a long day at work by tossing them in the pressure cooker with a little bit of stock and a sauce. I have a nice, healthy, home-cooked meal in 30 minutes.

The process of pressure cooking starts with boiling water or a water-based liquid (such as stock) inside a sealed pot. As the pot fills with steam, the pressure increases inside the pot until it reaches a set point. Due to the higher pressure, the water inside boils at a higher temperature, cooking most foods two to three times faster than other conventional methods, whether the food is immersed in the cooking liquid or not.

The shorter cook time in the pressure cooker also preserves vitamins and nutrients more than traditional cooking methods. One study published in the *Journal of Food Science* investigated vitamin C and sulforaphane (because its anticancer properties are of interest) retention in broccoli through various cooking methods. According to the abstract, boiling broccoli causes 34% loss of these nutrients, while steaming broccoli causes 22% loss of vitamin C, whereas microwaving and pressure cooking only experience a 10% loss. After boiling or steaming, sulforaphane was no longer detected in the broccoli, but after microwaving or pressure cooking, there was no loss.[1]

One common observation about pressure-cooked foods is that they seem "more flavorful." This is believed to be achieved by the Maillard reaction, where complex flavors are developed at higher temperatures. Also, by cooking in a sealed vessel, aromatic compounds that are normally boiled off are retained and the food has a chance to infuse better—or, perhaps it's a combination of the two.

Another benefit is that the pressure cooker uses less energy by cutting down cook time. It can also save money by tackling tougher, cheaper cuts of meat and allowing them to fall off the bone for melt-in-your-mouth tenderness in less time.

Frequently Asked Questions

Q: Cooking under pressure sounds dangerous. Is it?

A: These aren't your grandmother's pressure cookers! Pressure cooking and pressure cooking technology have been around for a long time and have come a long way. Both stovetop pressure cookers and electric pressure cookers have so many safety features built in and have been rigorously tested. As long as they're used properly and all safeguards are followed, they're perfectly safe.

Q: What's the difference between stovetop and electric pressure cookers?

---

1 F. Galgano, et al. "The Influence of Processing and Preservation on the Retention of Health-Promoting Compounds in Broccoli." *Journal of Food Science*, 72(2), 2007: S130-S135.

A: Stovetop pressure cookers require an external heat source, while electric pressure cookers are completely contained where the heating element is housed in the unit.

Electric pressure cookers have been packaged as multifunction appliances, where they may also work as a rice cooker, steamer, slow cooker, or yogurt maker depending on their programming. Essentially, several appliances can be replaced by one multifunction cooker. They're a little more sophisticated than their stovetop counterparts. However, they do cost more and are bulkier than the stovetop models.

Newer stovetop pressure cookers have two set pressures with a high operating pressure of 15 psi (compared to the 11.6 psi of some electric pressure cookers). The higher pressure means it gets hotter and cooks faster. You'll initially have to babysit a stovetop cooker while it comes up to pressure; once it seals that you turn down the heat to maintain the pressure. With an electric pressure cooker, after the lid is locked, the pressure release valve closed, and the pressure selected and time set, you can just walk away.

For the most part in this book, we'll be working with electric pressure cookers/multifunction cookers using the pressure cooker function only. However, if you have a stovetop pressure cooker, the recipes will work just as well. Once your stovetop pressure cooker has reached pressure via medium-high heat, turn down the heat and start timing. Set the time for about 10% less than the time required of the electric pressure cooker. For example, if the recipe requires 25 minutes under high pressure, then use 22½ minutes. But, as there are differences between stovetop pressure cooker models, as you learn more about your own pressure cooker, you'll need to adjust accordingly.

Q: I just unboxed my pressure cooker. Now what?

A: Read the manual. No, seriously. Especially if this is your first experience pressure cooking, get to know the parts of your pressure cooker, and go through the diagram with your pressure cooker in front of you. It's important to know what safety features are specific to your pressure cooker, as well as the safeguards. This way, when you're ready to use it, you'll know what to look for and make sure everything is in place before heating.

Then, perform the water test!

Q: What's the water test?

A: There are two reasons to do the water test: 1) to make sure that your pressure cooker seals up properly and everything is working; and 2) for you to become familiar with the general workings of the pressure cooker without worrying about ruining a dish.

Follow the water test procedure provided by your pressure cooker manual. If it doesn't have one you can try this method:

Make sure the silicone seal/gasket is in place and is seated properly. Add 3 cups of water in the inner stainless steel pot. Close and lock the lid. Set the pressure value to seal.

Set the pressure cooker to LOW PRESSURE cook for 2 minutes.

Once it has completed its cook time, QUICK RELEASE the pressure and *stay clear* of the venting hot steam.

Q: What can I cook with it?

A: Pressure cooking shines with anything that involves boiling or steaming and especially braising, which requires cooking for a long period of time. What's tricky is when you've got components of a dish that cook quicker than others because they're more delicate, but that's easily overcome by staggering the addition of ingredients and also by using the lower pressure function.

Q: I have my own recipe that I want to adapt in the pressure cooker. How do I do that?

A: As you use your pressure cooker more, you'll get an idea how fast certain foods cook. Try a few recipes to get an idea of cooking times and/or reference a similar recipe and use similar cook times. For example, if you have a favorite pulled pork recipe, see if you can adapt my Korean-Inspired Pulled Pork (page 146) to make it work with your ingredients in the pressure cooker. Soon you'll become so familiar that you'll be able to come up with recipes on the fly along with doneness preferences.

Q: Am I able to can in my electric pressure cooker?

A: In short, no. The USDA hasn't fully evaluated the safety of foods canned with electric pressure cookers, especially when it comes to low-acid foods such as meats and vegetables. It's uncertain with the lower pressures experienced with electric pressure cookers (versus stovetop pressure canners) that the temperature is high enough to properly process low-acid foods safely. If in doubt, check with your local university Extension Office in the US. If you're interested in preserving foods by canning for more information, you can download the USDA's *Complete Guide to Home Canning* from the National Center for Home Food Preservation website.

Tips for Using Your Pressure Cooker

While use and care of your pressure cooker will vary by brand, these are a few good practices to keep in mind.

Minimum/Maximum Liquid Amount

Check the operating manual for your pressure cooker for minimum liquid operating requirements. You may need to bump up the amount of water called for in a recipe, especially if the water is used for generating steam, such as where a recipe recommends to use the pressure cooker's steamer rack.

By the same token, don't overfill the pot. Overfilling may block the steam release or vent pipe. The maximum amount of liquid your pressure cooker can hold should also be mentioned in your manual, but it's usually no more than two-thirds of the capacity. (However, if you're cooking something that will generate a bit of "foam," such as beans or oats, half capacity is the upper limit for liquid.)

Venting

When the time comes to open up that release valve to vent the hot steam from the pressure cooker, whether it's a little or a lot, you'll want to be very careful, not just for your own safety but anyone else's, including any pets. You'll want to avoid venting near or underneath your cabinets too.

I keep my pressure cooker on the stove, so when the time comes to vent, I just turn on the overhead fan before releasing the pressure. Just be careful not to turn on any of your stove's heating elements.

There shouldn't be any liquid flowing/spewing from the vent pipe. The pressure cooker still may be too hot to let all the steam go at once, so let it slowly bleed for a few seconds, then stop. Repeat.

Just make sure not to fill the pot more than two-thirds full. Follow the safety instructions provided in your manual.

Cleaning

With most electric pressure cookers, there's an inner stainless steel cooking pot, sealing ring/gasket, pressure release valve (pressure limit valve), and vent pipe/float valve (which usually controls the locking pin). *If the instructions here differ from those in your pressure cooker's manual, be sure to follow the cleaning directions specific to your appliance.*

Wash the stainless steel inner pot with dish soap, soak off any stuck-on foods, and refrain from using a harsh abrasive. It may be dishwasher safe—just double check!

Remove the sealing ring/gasket from the lid and hand wash with hot soapy water. Be sure to dry it before reseating.

Wipe down the underside of the lid with a soapy dish cloth and rinse under water. Pay particular attention to the vent pipe/float valve and the pressure release valve, making sure that it's clean and unobstructed.

Remove the pressure release valve and make sure that it's also clean, then dry and replace it.

Never submerge the base of the pressure cooker in water. As the outside is usually brushed stainless steel, use a soft moist cloth to clean and dry with a soft towel.

A NOTE ON SILICONE SEALING RINGS

With some pressure cookers, the silicone sealing ring/gasket can absorb odors and/or discolor with regular use. Usually, as long as they're cleaned thoroughly, the odor shouldn't transfer to other foods and discoloration shouldn't affect its durability. In some cases, when going from cooking a savory dish, such as a curry, to a sweet dish, such as cheesecake or panna cotta, some cooks have observed that there is some transference of flavor. I suggest picking up a few extra rings and designating one for savory foods and the other for sweet.

CHAPTER 3

Let's Get Cooking!

Before we dive into the recipes, here are some helpful notes on handy tools, ingredients, electric pressure cooker instructions used in the recipes, nutritional information, and alternative suggestions.

Handy Tools

Here's a list of a few tools that I've found helpful for pressure cooking.

Flat wire steamer rack, stainless steel with wire feet: If it doesn't already come with your pressure cooker, it's a must! It keeps foods and containers out of the water and off of the hot pan when needed.

Heatproof ½-cup ramekins or canning jars: Perfect when making individual portions of cheesecake, panna cotta, and custard.

Immersion or "stick" blender: This is great for pureeing hot soups without taking them out of the pot to blend. They range in cost, but an inexpensive one works just fine. Other popular common uses are making homemade mayonnaise, smoothies, and butter coffee.

Japanese hot pot skimmer: This is a very fine mesh flat sieve that skims foams from stock with ease. In ketogenic cooking, the natural fats liberated by cooking certain grades/cuts of meat may be a little much.

These natural fats are good for the ketogenic diet, but may be a little in excess to your liking. Feel free to just skim some off.

Measuring cups and spoons: These are essential in every kitchen. It's handy to have a couple of sets of each, one for dry and another for wet ingredients, especially if you don't have a kitchen scale.

Kitchen scale(s): It takes the guesswork out of measuring volume and portion sizes. Pick a scale useful to your needs. I use one scale for larger amounts of up to 11 pounds (5kg) and another that specializes in small amounts down to 0.01g for spices and lighter foods that the larger scale can't weigh.

Kitchen thermometer: Instant-read thermometers are essential in every kitchen for determining the doneness of meats accurately and safely.

Sealing rings: Because sealing rings can sometimes pick up unwanted flavors or may become discolored over time, I suggest picking up a few extra rings and designating one for savory foods and the other for sweet. Refer to the Cleaning section on page 15 for more information.

Small or mini silicon mitts: I use these a lot. I use them to pull out the inner pot in addition to taking hot objects out of the pressure cooker. The smaller versions are easier to maneuver and pick up smaller objects without feeling clumsy.

Springform pan: Cheesecakes are a little easier to pop out of the pan and work well for Mexican Taco Lasagna (page 33) too.

Vegetable steamer basket: It's collapsible for easy storage but expandable to fit almost any pot size. Good for not only cooking cauliflower and broccoli florets in a flash, but also chicken wings.

Ingredients to Have on Hand

DIY vs premade spice blends and mixes: I'm all for using preblended spices and spice mixes, but I was having difficulty choosing a specific brand to recommend that everyone has access to. Rather than leaving some recipes in this book a mystery by not having the specific spice blend recommendation I went old-school and mixed my own. Now you too know exactly what spices are in each recipe.

But if you have favorite blends and mixes you gravitate to and wish to substitute with them, please do! Just approximate the total amount used in the recipe and use the same amount. (For example, if a recipe uses 3 tablespoons of total spices, use 3 tablespoons of the mix.) The exception is if the substituted blend is predominantly on the hot and spicy side. Then use it a little more sparingly, unless you like your food hot. Be sure to check the ingredient label for any sugars, starches, and fillers the premade spice mix may contain.

Fats and oils: For some recipes, a particular oil or fat is recommended for flavor or for higher smoke point for searing, for which I often suggest avocado oil. But for the most part the oils used in these recipes are interchangeable, and you can use a substitute if you have any particular preference or dietary requirement.

Fresh versus dried herbs: Fresh herbs are wonderful if they are available, but that's not always practical so it's dried spices to the rescue! Dried spices are two to three times more concentrated than fresh. If you're using dried spices instead of fresh and a recipe calls for 1 tablespoon of a fresh herb, use 1 teaspoon of the dried version.

Heavy cream: I use heavy cream (33 to 36%) whenever I can, and coconut milk with cream other times. I sometimes use them interchangeably. You could substitute with lower fat cream such as half-and-half. Just keep in mind the carb content usually increases as milk fat percentage goes down.

Liquid aminos: Liquid aminos is a soy product that's not fermented but is gluten free. It tastes like soy sauce but without the carbs. Tamari can also be used as a substitute, as it's made without wheat.

Sea salt versus table salt: I like to use sea salt of all kinds—smoked, flaked, coarse, spiced, and also pink. Not only does sea salt contain more minerals than table salt does, but it doesn't have things like sugar, potassium iodide, and sodium thiosulfate, which are common in regular commercial table salt.

Stock, broth, and water: Homemade stock or broth is ideal. You know exactly what goes in it and you can season it to your particular liking or purpose. Commercial stocks are good too; just read the label to make sure you know what you're getting. If you don't have any stock or broth handy and are using water from the tap, use cool water. Hot tap water can pick up contaminants from the water heater and pipes that dissolve more readily in hot water than cold, which could affect the taste of your dish.

Swerve, erythritol, and other sweeteners: I use Swerve, which is a natural sweetener that's a mix of erythritol and oligosaccharides that can be used as a one-to-one replacement for white sugar.

Erythritol itself is a sugar alcohol and a natural sweetener that is naturally occurring in some fruits. For most people, erythritol isn't fully absorbed nor retained by the body, which doesn't affect blood glucose levels. Because it's not retained by the body, it hasn't been included in the nutrition value calculations. Unlike other sugar alcohols such as maltitol, which can cause stomach upset, erythritol does not have such side effects. It doesn't have an aftertaste, but some have experienced a "cooling" sensation on the tongue.

Stevia (steviol glycosides) is a natural sweetener from the leaves of the stevia plant that is 150 times sweeter than granulated sugar. Like erythritol, it has minimal effects on blood glucose levels. It can, however, have a bitter aftertaste.

Xylitol is another naturally occurring sweetener and sugar alcohol. It's found in small amounts in fruits and vegetables. It is low on the glycemic index scale and has a minimal effect on blood glucose levels.

It is, however, extremely harmful to dogs and can even be fatal, so use with caution.

It is quite common to use a couple of alternative sweeteners in tandem to offset or counteract the aftertaste of each other, which is why you'll see the use of two sweeteners in some of the recipes here.

Xanthan gum and other thickeners: In a few recipes, I've mentioned using xanthan gum. It's a gluten-free, low-carb thickener and emulsifier. Some sauces are nicer when they've got a thicker texture and have a better mouthfeel. To use xanthan gum, simply sprinkle it over your sauce and whisk it in. It thickens up pretty quickly while whisking. Keep sprinkling and whisking until you reach a desired consistency. Just be wary not to use too much, as the consistency can go "slimy."

How to Use an Electric Pressure Cooker

I'm the proud owner of two Instant Pots, the DUO60 and the Smart. I've also exchanged one and given another away so technically I've had four! I've been cooking with the Instant Pot for about two-and-a-half years now. Both the Instant Pots have a 6-quart capacity, and the recipes in this book were created using one or both of these workhorses. I don't know what I'd do without them now—they've made cooking so much easier.

These recipes can be made in any pressure cooker. Manufacturers of electric pressure cookers are different, as are their food-specific heating profiles. Rather than referencing the "POULTRY" or "SOUP" function, I've tried to keep it as generic as possible for all models by just referring to a "HIGH PRESSURE" setting for a specific amount of time. But cooking times may vary slightly if your pressure cooker differs in size or the pressure/heat specifications are different.

Pressure is created in pressure cookers by boiling water in a sealed container. As the water evaporates, it fills the container with steam. The more steam generated, the higher the pressure and the higher the temperature inside the container.

Primarily, pressure is measured in pounds per square inch, which is abbreviated as psi. Other parts of the world use kilopascals, which is abbreviated as kPa. On some pressure cookers, one can select a high or low pressure setting. With others, one may have the versatility of 5 or 6 pressure settings to select from. On the electric pressure cookers, there aren't any gauges to actually check pressure. Some older stovetop pressure cookers and pressure canners are equipped with a gauge to monitor pressure.

These are the cooking instructions (and what they mean) with reference to the pressure cooker, used in these recipes. You may not see all instructions in all recipes.

Prepare the pot: This draws your attention that you should heat up the pressure cooker or add some water and put a steam rack in to get ready.

Set the pressure cooker to SAUTÉ: The SAUTÉ, OPEN SEAR, SEAR, or BROWN function will heat up the element nice and hot for you to sauté or sear your food. (Tip: If you want to preheat the water before pressurizing, this button will do it for you.) The regular temperature the Instant Pot uses for this setting is: 275°F to 300°F (135°C to 150°C).

Set the pressure cooker to SAUTÉ, higher setting: With some pressure cookers, you can increase the searing/browning temperature. When you see this instruction, just bump up the temperature on your appliance. If you don't have this function on your cooker, not to worry—the regular temperature will still get you the results you need. The higher sauté temperature the Instant Pot uses is 350°F to 410°F (175°C to 210°C).

Cover with the lid and lock: Cover the pressure cooker and lock the lid into place, making sure it is secure. *Make sure the sealing ring is clean and seated properly beforehand.*

SEAL the pressure release valve: The pressure release valve (or pressure limit valve) is a safety valve that releases or holds the steam in the pot depending on the valve's position or orientation, whether it's opened or closed. *Make sure the valve isn't blocked from the top or the underside every time you use the pressure cooker.* Seal the pressure release valve, to seal or toggle to the closed position for pressurizing. Get ready to pressurize!

Set to HIGH PRESSURE and cook for X minutes: Set your pressure cooker to cook at high pressure for the number of minutes indicated in the recipe. Some cookers have a default high pressure set. For the Instant Pot, high pressure is automatically set at 10.2 to 11.6 psi (70 to 80 kPa).

Set to HIGH PRESSURE and cook for 0 minutes: This isn't a typo! There are times when some or all of the foods in the pressure cooker can overcook really fast, such as in some vegetables, fish, and shellfish dishes. To reap the benefits of infusing flavors but not overcooking, the pressure cooker is just brought up to pressure then quickly released.

Set to LOW PRESSURE and cook for X minutes: Set your pressure cooker to cook at a low pressure for the number of minutes indicated in the recipe. If you are lucky and can adjust the pressure, use 5.8 to 7.2 psi, which is the default low pressure on the Instant Pot. Please refer to your cooker's manual. This setting is good for foods, such as small dice zucchini or finely shredded cabbage, that need to be cooked for a little longer but are overcooked within seconds under high pressure.

Set to WARM: Set your cooker to the WARM or KEEP WARM function. This is for when you just need a little bit of heat to keep things nice and toasty!

Then QUICK RELEASE: After the cook time has been reached, open up the pressure release valve (or pressure limit valve) from sealing to venting to let the steam escape and bring the pressure down rapidly. For some cookers it's also known as RAPID RELEASE. Let 'er rip! Just steer clear of the hot steam evacuating the pot. I use the pot underneath the kitchen fan and turn it on just before releasing the pressure. Keep the fan on when opening the pressure cooker lid. After unlocking the lid, lift it up slightly and tilt it away from you.

Then NATURAL RELEASE: After the cook time has been reached, just let the pressure cooker come down in pressure on its own. You don't have to do a thing. Sometimes the food needs more time to cook, but in some cases where the pot is full, it needs to depressurize slowly, rather than getting "shocked" in the quick release pressure drop.

Then MANUAL RELEASE PRESSURE after X minutes: After the cook time has been reached, wait the number of minutes indicated before manually releasing the pressure. Some foods just need a little more time to cook or settle before releasing the pressure.

Nutrition Facts

The nutritional information for each recipe has been provided as a reference guideline and is approximate for those who keep track of their individual macronutrient (fat, protein, and carbohydrate/net carbohydrate) and caloric intake.

Products can differ not only from country to country but even from one producer to the next.

If you're counting macros strictly, I suggest that you weigh all ingredients and use the product information provided on labels to calculate the nutrition data for accuracy.

The nutritional information has been compiled using Nutrifox and manually from manufacturer product labels and the United States Department of Agriculture, Agricultural Research Service, and National Nutrient Database for Standard Reference Release.

In the recipes, you'll see:

Nutrition Facts (amount per serving)	
Energy (calories)	351
Fat	26.3g
Protein	21.9g
Total Carbohydrates	7.7g
Fiber	2.5g
Net Carbohydrates	5.2g

Macronutrient Breakdown	
Fat	67%
Protein	25%
Carbs	8%

Breaking it down, the nutritional information provided is per serving size. In the example, it's per ½ cup serving size. Serving size was determined by either evenly dividing up the portions or by using 4-ounce (113g) protein portions. In each recipe, serving size will be listed along with yield. Using this as a guideline, you can adjust your intake accordingly by increasing or decreasing your portion size.

Energy is the amount of calories per serving, which in this example is 351 calories (kcal). The conversion from the weight of the macronutrient to energy is as follows:

1g fat = 9 calories

1g carbohydrates = 4 calories

1g protein = 4 calories

Fat is the amount of fat contained in the serving = 26.3g

Protein is the amount of protein in the serving = 21.9g

Net Carbohydrates = the amount of *total carbohydrates* (7.7g) - *fiber* (2.5g) = 5.2g

Macronutrient breakdown is the percentage of calories broken down into their macronutrient components. Some people use this as a guide for their macronutrient intake. Of the 351 calories, 67% of those calories are fat, 25% are protein, and 8% are total carbohydrates. I've kept the percentage of carbs in terms of total carbohydrates and not net carbohydrates, as I know there are some ketogenic dieters that look at total carbohydrates for their calculations.

Please note that nutritional values haven't been included for broth or stock. Short of having these tested by a lab, I haven't been able to source a reliable and accurate way of determining the nutritional information for stock or broth. All the components used to make it (vegetables, bones with scraps of meat, etc.) are discarded, and fat may or may not be scraped off. What is left is an infusion of these elements, leaving minimal macronutrients, and I've seen them range from 30 to 40 calories or as much as 80 calories per cup.

Variations

Where possible, alternative suggestions, variations, and different ideas were included for most recipes. These are meant to help you see the possibility in the dishes. Cooking can be creative and inspiring. The more you learn and try different things, the more likely you'll discover new favorites and be inspired to create your own recipes.

Recipe Icons

While skimming through recipes, look for these symbols as a guide:

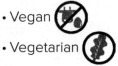

- Dairy Free
- Peanut and Nut Free
- Egg Free
- Vegan
- Vegetarian

CHAPTER 4
Beef

Beef Stock

For a rich beef stock, it's always best to roast the bones before letting them simmer away. My dear friend Peggy is known to roast bones for stock overnight in her electric roaster, and it brings about a really nice and robust stock. If you can't easily find beef marrow bones, just ask your butcher to save you some.

MAKES approximately 3 quarts or 12 (1-cup) servings

3 pounds (1.3kg) beef bones, preferably marrow bones

½ teaspoon (3g) sea salt

pinch black pepper

1 medium onion, halved, skin on

2 large carrots, halved

3 celery stalks, halved

1 tablespoon (18g) salt

1 tablespoon (9g) whole black peppercorns

1 tablespoon (15g) apple cider vinegar

1. Preheat the oven to 375°F.

2. Sprinkle salt and a little pepper on the beef bones.

3. Line a shallow roasting pan with foil.

4. Place the bones in the pan roast for a minimum of 30 minutes.

PREPARE THE POT

5. Add the bones, onion, carrots, celery, salt, peppercorns, and apple cider vinegar to the pot.

6. Fill with cool water to 1 inch from the max-fill line.

7. Close and lock lid. SEAL the pressure release valve.

8. Set to HIGH PRESSURE and cook for 75 minutes.

9. Then let the pot NATURAL RELEASE the pressure, about 15 minutes.

10. Remove the bones, onions, carrots, and celery. Strain the stock if necessary.

11. Let cool and skim off some or all of the fat, if desired.

12. If you're not using the stock immediately, store in the fridge for a few days. Or, for longer storage, place in a Ziploc bag, remove the air, and place it in the freezer for up to 3 months.

VARIATION: Depending on what you plan to do with the stock, add bay leaves and other aromatic herbs, like rosemary and fennel seed.

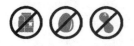

Nutrition facts and macronutrient breakdowns are not included for stocks and broths (see page 26).

Beef Pho

In my town, we have a little restaurant that makes the best beef pho broth. It simmers overnight and I crave it when I'm sick. Unfortunately, I can't have too much of it as it will knock me out of ketosis. I wanted to create a broth that could be made in less time and be keto-friendly. This recipe makes about 10 cups of broth, depending on the size of your cooker. It freezes well for those times when you have a craving for pho or are looking to drink a tasty electrolyte replenisher. Some butchers will cut the thinly sliced beef you'll need for pho for you, but you may have to order a minimum quantity.

MAKES about 10 cups or 6 (1½-cup) servings

2 teaspoons (5g) whole coriander seeds

1 cinnamon stick or ½ teaspoon (2.6g) ground cinnamon

4 whole cloves

2 whole star anise

2 whole black cardamom pods (optional)

4 pounds (1.8kg) beef bones

2 medium onions, halved, skin on

3 inches (7.6 cm) fresh ginger, halved lengthwise, skin on

2 tablespoons (30mL) fish sauce

5 teaspoons (20g) Swerve sweetener or erythritol

1 tablespoon (18g) salt

4 ounces (114g) thinly sliced beef sirloin per serving

bean sprouts, to serve

cilantro, to serve

jalapeño slices, to serve

Thai basil, to serve

shirataki noodles, to serve

limes, to serve

1. Mix together the coriander, cinnamon, cloves, star anise, and cardamom. Set aside.

PREPARE THE POT

2. Place the beef bones in the pot and fill with water until it just covers them.

3. Close and lock lid. SEAL the pressure release valve.

4. Set to HIGH PRESSURE and cook for 7 minutes.

5. Then carefully RELEASE PRESSURE after 1 to 2 minutes.

6. While the bones are parboiling, char the onions and ginger by placing them on a cookie sheet under the oven's broiler for 3 to 4 minutes or on a gas stove element for 2 to 3 minutes, until the surface is charred. Set aside.

7. Remove the beef bones from the pot. Rinse under cool tap water, removing any grayish residue.

8. When they're cool enough to handle, use your hands to lightly rub off any loose proteins and rinse again.

9. Remove any marrow with a butter knife or spoon. Set the bones aside.

10. Wash the pressure cooker pot and lid, if there are any solid bits left on the lid.

11. Re-insert the pot.

12. Place the beef bones, onions, ginger, fish sauce, Swerve or erythritol, salt, and the spice mixture in the pot.

13. Fill with cool water to 1 inch from the max-fill line.

14. Close and lock lid.

15. Set to HIGH PRESSURE and cook for 75 minutes.

16. Then carefully RELEASE the pressure after 5 minutes.

17. Remove the bones, onions, ginger, and spices, and skim off any protein solids. Strain if necessary.

18. To serve, place 4 ounces of rare sliced beef at the bottom of a bowl. Ladle 1½ cups of fresh hot broth from the pressure cooker over the top. Garnish with bean sprouts, cilantro, jalapeño slices, Thai basil, shirataki noodles, and lime, as desired.

VARIATION: Try making the broth with pork or even lamb. The parboiling step at the beginning may not be necessary when using other proteins.

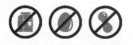

Nutrition Facts	
(amount per serving)	
Energy (calories)	268
Fat	16.3g
Protein	25.2g
Total Carbohydrates	2.5g
Fiber	0g
Net Carbohydrates	2.5g

Macronutrient Breakdown	
Fat	55%
Protein	38%
Carbs	4%

Mexican Taco Lasagna

This was fun to make and best of all it was tasty! If you've got a deep springform pan (3 inches deep), you can play around with lots of low-carb friendly fillings in the layers as long as it's not too runny. I used a 2½-inch-deep pan for this recipe and it just fit! You don't have to put it under the broiler at the end; just add the cheese on top before covering it with foil. I just like the browned, melting, cheesy goodness on top.

MAKES 6 (1-slice) servings

Taco Spices

1½ teaspoons (3g) ground cumin

2 teaspoons (2.5g) ancho chile powder

¼ teaspoon (0.5g) red chile flakes

¼ teaspoon (0.3g) dried oregano

½ teaspoon (1g) paprika

1½ (9g) teaspoons salt

½ teaspoon (1.4g) ground black pepper

¼ teaspoon (0.5g) cayenne pepper (optional)

Cheese Mixture

1 cup (250g) cottage cheese, 2%, drained

2 tablespoons (18g) prepared salsa

1 egg, lightly beaten

1½ cups (180g) shredded cheddar cheese

Lasagna

2 tablespoons (30mL) avocado oil or olive oil

½ cup (55g) chopped onion

1 pound (454g) ground beef

2 cloves garlic, minced

4 low-carb tortillas (8¾oz, 248g)

½ cup (60g) shredded cheddar cheese

sour cream, to serve

sliced black olives, to serve

diced fresh tomatoes, to serve

jalapeños, fresh or canned, to serve

hot sauce, to serve

shredded lettuce, to serve

chopped green onions, to serve

guacamole, to serve

salsa, to serve

1. Mix the spices together and set aside.

2. Drain any excess liquid from the cottage cheese. Mix in the salsa, egg, and cheddar cheese. Set aside.

PREPARE THE POT

3. Set the pressure cooker to SAUTÉ.

4. Once hot, add the olive oil or avocado oil.

5. Add half the onion and sauté until translucent, about 1½ minutes.

6. Add the ground beef and brown.

7. Add the rest of onion and the garlic, then stir in the spice mix.

8. Drain off the fat, and turn off pressure cooker.

9. Cut the tortillas to size. The best way to do this is to take the closed ring from the springform pan and place it on top of the tortilla. Then with a small utility knife, trace the inside of the ring, cutting the tortilla. Repeat with the other three tortillas.

10. Reassemble the springform pan and wrap the bottom in foil. This prevents extra moisture from seeping in through the bottom.

11. Place one tortilla in the bottom of the pan. Spoon one-third of the meat mixture onto the tortilla and spread evenly.

12. Remix the cheese mix, if necessary, and spoon one third on top of the meat mixture and spread evenly.

13. Place a second tortilla on top, and repeat the layers, finishing with the fourth tortilla on top.

14. Cover the springform pan with foil.

15. Wash the pressure cooker insert.

16. Add 1½ cups of water to the pot, place flat steamer rack in the pot and a foil sling if needed.

17. Carefully place the springform pan on rack.

18. Close lid and lock. SEAL the pressure valve.

19. Set to HIGH PRESSURE and cook for 12 minutes.

20. Then MANUAL RELEASE PRESSURE after 1 minute.

21. Take the springform pan out of the pressure cooker and place it on a cookie sheet.

22. Remove the foil top, and sprinkle on the shredded cheddar cheese.

23. Place in the oven under the broiler for 2 to 3 minutes, or until the cheese is bubbling.

24. Remove from the oven and let cool for about a minute.

25. Run a knife along the inside of the springform pan ring. Cut the lasagna into 6 pieces. Remove the springform pan ring.

26. Serve with your favorite taco condiments and toppings, especially sour cream and guacamole to add more good keto fats in.

VARIATIONS: Substituting ground chicken or turkey instead of beef would work really well. Or, for something a little different use cooked shredded beef, pork, or chicken. Try a jalapeño pepper–Colby Jack cheese mixed in or instead of cheddar. Change it up a little: Mix the cheese with drained and squeezed cooked spinach and make it the middle layer, with the meat-only layers on the top and bottom.

Nutrition Facts	
(amount per serving)	
Energy (calories)	537
Fat	37g
Protein	33.7g
Total Carbohydrates	17.5g
Fiber	9.6g
Net Carbohydrates	7.9g

Macronutrient Breakdown	
Fat	62%
Protein	25%
Carbs	13%

Barbecue Beef Boneless Short Ribs

While this recipe is ready in just 5 minutes, if you have the time to let it cook for 35 to 40 minutes, the fat on the short ribs will melt and the meat will almost fall apart. Simply heaven! Add the xanthan gum for a thicker sauce, or feel free to omit it altogether. You can easily make the sauce ahead of time (even a day or two) to let the flavors mingle; just refrigerate until you're ready.

MAKES 6 (1-cup) servings

Sauce

1½ cups (375mL) sugar-free ketchup

¼ cup (60mL) liquid aminos, tamari, or soy sauce

1 teaspoon (5mL) Worcestershire sauce

1 tablespoon (15g) sriracha

1 tablespoon (15mL) apple cider vinegar

2 teaspoons (12g) salt

1 teaspoon (5g) Swerve sweetener or erythritol

¼ teaspoon (0.5g) ground ginger

2 cloves garlic, finely minced

Short Ribs

2¾ pounds (1.25kg) boneless beef short ribs, cut into 1½-inch cubes

1 teaspoon (6g) salt

½ teaspoon (1.5g) freshly ground pepper

2 tablespoons (30mL) avocado oil

½ cup (70g) chopped onion

1½ cups (375mL) beef stock, divided

7 white mushrooms, quartered

½ teaspoon (1.2g) xanthan gum (optional)

1. Whisk all the sauce ingredients together. Set aside.

2. Sprinkle salt and pepper on beef cubes.

PREPARE THE POT

3. Set the pressure cooker to SAUTÉ, higher setting.

4. Once the pot is hot, add the avocado oil.

5. Brown the meat on all sides in batches, about 2 to 3 minutes per side. Remove from the pot once browned.

6. Add the onion to the oil and sauté for 1 minute.

7. Add ½ cup of the beef stock, and stir to deglaze the pot.

8. Add the sauce and the remaining 1 cup of beef stock.

9. Return the beef to the pot, along with any drippings.

10. Close lid and lock. SEAL the pressure release valve.

11. Set to HIGH PRESSURE and cook for 5 minutes.

12. Then QUICK RELEASE after 5 minutes.

13. Add the mushrooms.

14. Set to LOW PRESSURE and cook for 1 minute.

15. Then QUICK RELEASE.

16. Sprinkle in the xanthan gum, if using, and stir to thicken.

VARIATION: Since the sauce has a bold flavor, any cut of beef would work best, but I can imagine cooking pork ribs in this sauce as well.

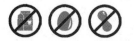

Nutrition Facts	
(amount per serving)	
Energy (calories)	447
Fat	28.5g
Protein	41g
Total Carbohydrates	6.1g
Fiber	0.03g
Net Carbohydrates	6.1g

Macronutrient Breakdown	
Fat	57%
Protein	37%
Carbs	6%

Top Round Roast

The top round cut is known as "inside round" in Canada, but it's the same cut of meat. When it's cut into steaks, they're known as top round steaks, London Broil, or breakfast steak. The recipe calls for one stick of butter, but you can easily add another half or even a second stick, as this cut typically doesn't have a lot of fat. This recipe is quite versatile, and you can shred the meat and serve it over Cauliflower Mash (page 186), or slice the roast into steaks after the initial one hour of cooking. It's also good served with a side of green beans and topped with sliced avocado.

MAKES 8 (1-cup) servings

2 tablespoons (30mL) ghee or avocado oil

2 to 3 teaspoons (12 to 18g) sea salt

2½ pounds (1.1kg) top round roast

1 medium onion, chopped

3 cloves garlic, minced

1 cup (250mL) beef or vegetable stock

½ teaspoon (1.4g) coarsely ground pepper

1 stick (½ cup, 110g) salted butter

1 tablespoon (1.3g) dried rosemary

1 tablespoon (1.3g) dried thyme

1 bay leaf

PREPARE THE POT

1. Set the pressure cooker to SAUTÉ, high setting.

2. Once hot, add the ghee or avocado oil.

3. Sprinkle salt all over the roast.

4. Brown the meat on all sides, approximately 2 to 3 minutes per side, then remove from the pot and set aside.

5. Add the onion and garlic to the pot, and sauté for 1 minute.

6. Add the beef stock and stir to deglaze the pot.

7. Add the pepper.

8. Add the roast back in, along with any drippings.

9. Add the butter on top.

10. Close lid and lock. SEAL the pressure release valve.

11. Set to HIGH PRESSURE and cook for 60 minutes.

12. Then QUICK RELEASE.

13. Take the roast out and cut into 4 to 5 large pieces. Return to the pot.

14. Add the rosemary, thyme, and bay leaf.

15. Set to HIGH PRESSURE and cook for 15 minutes.

16. Then QUICK RELEASE.

17. Shred the meat and season to taste.

VARIATIONS: Instead of using thyme, rosemary, and bay leaf for seasonings, use liquid aminos, Worcestershire sauce, and chile paste with a little sesame oil. Or use 1 cup (2 sticks) of butter, 2 more cloves of garlic, and regular prepared yellow mustard or Dijon mustard. For a spicier version, add a can of drained jalapeños and/or a can of chipotle peppers with adobo sauce before cooking for the last 15 minutes.

Nutrition Facts	
(amount per serving)	
Energy (calories)	366
Fat	25.7g
Protein	30.5g
Total Carbohydrates	2g
Fiber	0.4g
Net Carbohydrates	1.6g

Macronutrient Breakdown	
Fat	64%
Protein	34%
Carbs	2%

Top Round Roast Stew

Some have said that eating ketogenic can be expensive. Look for items on sale and try to prepare them in different ways. I came across a great sale for top round roast. It's quite a lean roast, so bacon helps in bumping up the fats a little. This stew is also packed with a bunch of great veggies. Feel free to change it up!

MAKES 8 (1¼-cup) servings

Spices

2 tablespoons (15.2g) paprika

1½ tablespoons (6.5g) dried oregano

2 teaspoons (6g) ground cumin

½ teaspoon (1.5g) ground chipotle pepper (for more heat, add another ½ to 1 teaspoon)

1 tablespoon (18g) sea salt

Stew

3 strips bacon, cut into ½-inch pieces

1 teaspoon (6g) salt

2½ pounds (1.2kg) top round roast, cubed

1 medium onion, chopped

2 cloves garlic, minced

1 cup (250mL) beef or vegetable stock

1 (28oz, 796mL) can diced tomatoes, drained

2½ cups (175g) broccoli florets

8 white mushrooms, sliced

3 cups (285g) cubed zucchini, skin on

4 cups (373g) cubed eggplant, skin on

sliced avocado, to serve

sour cream, to serve

1. Mix the spices together and set aside.

PREPARE THE POT

2. Set the pressure cooker to SAUTÉ.

3. Once hot, add the bacon pieces. Stir a little to warm up and slightly crisp the bacon, about 4 minutes.

4. Sprinkle salt on beef pieces, then brown the beef in batches and remove.

5. Add the onion and sauté until translucent, about a minute, then add the garlic and stir for 30 seconds.

6. Add the beef or vegetable stock, and stir to deglaze the pot.

7. Add the tomatoes. Stir in the spices.

8. Close lid and lock. SEAL the pressure release valve.

9. Set to HIGH PRESSURE and cook for 15 to 20 minutes.

10. Then QUICK RELEASE.

11. Stir in the broccoli, mushrooms, zucchini, and eggplant.

12. Set to HIGH PRESSURE and cook for 1 to 2 minutes, or set to LOW PRESSURE and cook for 15 minutes.

13. Then MANUAL RELEASE PRESSURE after 1 minute.

14. Ladle into bowls and serve with sliced avocado and sour cream, if desired.

VARIATION: Use can use a fattier cut of beef or stewing beef, but you'll need to cook it for about 20 minutes longer as these cuts tend to be tougher. You can cut back on the added fat (bacon), if you prefer, or just keep it in.

Nutrition Facts	
(amount per serving)	
Energy (calories)	355
Fat	21.6g
Protein	39g
Total Carbohydrates	12.7g
Fiber	5.2g
Net Carbohydrates	7.5g

Macronutrient Breakdown	
Fat	48.7%
Protein	39%
Carbs	12.7%

Prime Rib Roast

It is such a treat when I can find a sale on prime rib roast. Traditionally it takes hours to do a roast in the oven, but by using the pressure cooker, it doesn't have to be a Sunday to make a decadent meal like this. Unless you're feeding a small crowd, there will be leftovers for a few lunches. This recipe also makes its own au jus (sauce)—flavorful drippings from the roast cascade into the beef stock and intermingle with the garlic and onion. It's delicious served with Hickory Alfredo Cauliflower Mash (page 188).

MAKES 6 (6-ounce) servings, about ½ rib each

Rub Spices

2 tablespoons (15.2g) paprika

2 teaspoons (12g) sea salt

½ teaspoon (1.4g) black pepper

2 teaspoons (2g) dried thyme

2 teaspoons (2g) dried rosemary

2 teaspoons (1.4g) dried basil

⅛ teaspoon (0.22g) cayenne pepper

1 teaspoon (2g) ground mustard

Prime Rib

1½ cups (375mL) beef or vegetable stock

2 cloves garlic, halved lengthwise

1 medium onion, halved

5 pounds (2.3kg) bone-in prime rib roast, at room temperature

salt

freshly ground pepper

1. Mix together the spices for the rub and set aside.

PREPARE THE POT

2. Add the stock, garlic, and onion to the pot.

3. Place a flat wire steaming rack in the pot.

4. Pat the roast dry, then pat it all over with the spice rub mixture.

5. Set the roast on the rack with the bones to one side.

6. Close the lid and lock. SEAL the pressure valve.

7. Set to HIGH PRESSURE and cook for 30 to 35 minutes.

8. Then MANUAL RELEASE PRESSURE after 1 minute.

9. Take the roast out and check the internal temperature with a kitchen thermometer. Aim for 5 to 10°F below the desired doneness temperature as the temperature will rise while resting. For rare, aim for about 115°F for a final temperature of 120 to 125°F. For medium rare, aim for about 125°F for a final temperature of 130 to 135°F.

10. Remove the roast from the pot and let it sit covered with foil to rest for 15 to 30 minutes.

11. While the roast is resting, prepare the au jus.

12. Remove the wire rack, garlic, and onion from the pot.

13. Skim off about half the fat, and whisk in salt and pepper to taste.

14. Slice the roast and serve with the jus.

VARIATION: For a little more complex jus, after skimming off the fat, add either 1 tablespoon dry red wine (this would add 1g carb) or 1 tablespoon liquid aminos and a sprig of fresh rosemary. Cover and set the pot to SAUTÉ for 2 to 3 minutes. Remove the rosemary sprig and season with salt and pepper to taste.

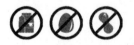

Nutrition Facts	
(amount per serving)	
Energy (calories)	608
Fat	54g
Protein	27.7g
Total Carbohydrates	0.8g
Fiber	0.5g
Net Carbohydrates	0.3g

Macronutrient Breakdown	
Fat	80%
Protein	18%
Carbs	0.5%

Rib Eye Au Jus

Rib eye steak has one of the best fat-to-protein ratios for the keto diet. It's such a treat to have. This is the perfect dish to serve over Hickory Alfredo Cauliflower Mash (page 188).

MAKES 4 (4-ounce) servings

2 tablespoons (27mL) coconut oil

1 pound (454g) rib eye steak, cut into 1-inch cubes

1 cup (250mL) beef stock

¼ cup (60mL) liquid aminos

1 teaspoon (5mL) Worcestershire sauce

6 medium mushrooms, quartered

½ teaspoon (2.8g) freshly ground pepper, plus more for seasoning

¼ teaspoon (1.5g) sea salt, plus more for seasoning

¼ teaspoon xanthan gum (optional)

PREPARE THE POT

1. Set the pressure cooker to SAUTÉ, high setting.

2. Once hot, add the coconut oil.

3. Sprinkle the meat with salt and pepper

4. Brown the meat in the hot oil, in batches if necessary. Then remove and set aside.

5. Add the stock and stir to deglaze the pot.

6. Add the liquid aminos, Worcestershire sauce, mushrooms, pepper, and sea salt.

7. Add the meat back in, along with any drippings.

8. Close the lid and lock. SEAL the pressure valve.

9. Set to HIGH PRESSURE and cook for 5 minutes.

10. Then MANUAL RELEASE PRESSURE after 2 minutes.

11. Remove the meat.

12. If desired, sprinkle xanthan gum over the sauce and whisk through to thicken.

13. Pour the sauce over the rib eye to serve.

VARIATION: The combination of liquid aminos and Worcestershire lends itself really well to beef, bison, and ostrich. Use other cuts of meat with this combination. Start with a 15- to 20-minute cook time for regular cuts of meat and 30 to 40 minutes for tougher cuts.

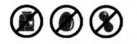

Nutrition Facts	
(amount per serving)	
Energy (calories)	362
Fat	29.6g
Protein	23g
Total Carbohydrates	2.4g
Fiber	0.4g
Net Carbohydrates	2g

Macronutrient Breakdown	
Fat	73%
Protein	25%
Carbs	2%

Corned Beef Brisket with Cabbage

These days you can find corned beef brisket at your local butcher that's already packed in a brine and has been curing for a few days. Normally it takes hours of cooking for the brisket to soften, but it takes much less time using the pressure cooker.

MAKES 5 (4½-ounce) servings

1 cup (250mL) beef stock

2½ pounds (1 kg) beef brisket packed in brine

1 medium onion, sliced

¼ head green cabbage, cored and shredded

2 teaspoons (2g) caraway seeds

sour cream, to serve

chopped green onions, to serve

PREPARE THE POT

1. Pour the beef stock into the pot.

2. Remove the brisket from the package and place it in the pot along with the brine.

3. Close the lid and lock. SEAL the pressure valve.

4. Set to HIGH PRESSURE and cook for 60 minutes.

5. Then QUICK RELEASE.

6. Remove the brisket from the pot.

7. Spread the onion and cabbage in the pot and sprinkle caraway seeds over the top.

8. Slice the beef brisket across the grain into 1-inch-thick pieces.

9. Place the sliced beef over the cabbage.

10. Close the lid and lock. SEAL the pressure valve.

11. Set to HIGH PRESSURE for 6 minutes.

12. Then QUICK RELEASE.

13. Serve the brisket with the cabbage and top with sour cream and chopped green onions, if desired.

VARIATION: Rather than just cabbage alone, put together a mix of shredded green and red cabbage with a little bit of grated carrot, and mix in some thinly sliced bok choy.

Nutrition Facts (amount per serving)	
Energy (calories)	381
Fat	27.9g
Protein	23.9g
Total Carbohydrates	8.3g
Fiber	3.3g
Net Carbohydrates	5g

Macronutrient Breakdown	
Fat	66%
Protein	25%
Carbs	8%

Italian Meatballs

Normally for recipes using ground beef, I'll use regular ground (70/30) for the extra fat. This recipe uses ground pork as well, so I've called for lean ground beef to cut back on the total fat, but I encourage using a higher percentage fat beef whenever you can. Serve over zoodles, shirataki noodles, kelp noodles, spaghetti squash, or any other low-carb noodle.

MAKES about 6 (3-meatball) servings

Meatball Mixture

1 pound (454g) lean (83/17) ground beef

1 pound (454g) ground pork

½ medium onion, finely chopped

3 cloves garlic, finely minced

1 teaspoon (0.3g) dried basil

½ teaspoon (1.3g) red chile flakes

2 eggs, lightly beaten

½ cup (50g) finely grated Parmesan cheese

1½ teaspoons (9g) salt

½ teaspoon (1.4g) ground pepper

Sauce

2 tablespoons (27.2g) coconut oil

½ medium onion, chopped (optional)

1 clove garlic, minced (optional)

½ cup (125mL) beef stock

1 (28oz, 796mL) can diced tomatoes with liquid

1. Combine the ingredients for the meatball mixture in a large bowl and mix well. It works much better using damp hands. Measure out 2 tablespoons of mixture and roll into a ball. Repeat with the rest of the mixture. Makes about 18 meatballs.

PREPARE THE POT

2. Set the pressure cooker to SAUTÉ, high setting.

3. Once hot, add the coconut oil to melt.

4. Brown meatballs in batches, remove, and set aside.

5. Add the onion, if using, to the pot and sauté until translucent. Stir in the garlic, if using.

6. Pour in the stock and stir to deglaze the pot.

7. Stir in the tomatoes.

8. Add the meatballs back in, along with any drippings.

9. Close the lid and lock. SEAL the pressure valve.

10. Set to HIGH PRESSURE and cook for 12 minutes.

11. Then QUICK RELEASE.

VARIATIONS: Instead of using Parmesan cheese, use Asiago or Romano cheese, or a mix. Leaner meats such as ground chicken and turkey can be used, but be sure to add in some fat such as lard or bacon fat for moisture.

Nutrition Facts	
(amount per serving)	
Energy (calories)	461
Fat	2.2g
Protein	34.5g
Total Carbohydrates	7.8g
Fiber	3.1g
Net Carbohydrates	4.7g

Macronutrient Breakdown	
Fat	63%
Protein	30%
Carbs	7%

Kare-Kare
(Filipino Oxtail Stew)

I have fond memories of this dish from when I was growing up. It would take the greater part of the day to cook the oxtail to until the meat fell off the bone. We didn't have it often, but it was one of my favorites. Now with the pressure cooker it takes only a couple of hours to make and is just as delicious.

MAKES 5 (½-cup) servings

2 tablespoons (30mL) avocado oil

2¾ pounds (1.25kg) beef oxtail

1 cup (160g) chopped onion

3 cloves garlic, minced

1 cup (250mL) beef or vegetable stock

¼ cup (100g) natural peanut butter

1 tablespoon (18g) sea salt

½ teaspoon (1.4g) ground pepper

3½ cups (300g) cubed Chinese eggplant

12 ounces (340g) Chinese long beans or string beans, cut into thirds

1 tablespoon (15mL) fish sauce (optional)

PREPARE THE POT

1. Set the pressure cooker to SAUTÉ, high setting.

2. When hot, add the avocado oil.

3. Brown the oxtail in batches, then remove and set aside.

4. Sauté the onion and garlic until the onions are translucent, about a minute.

5. Pour the stock into the pot and stir to deglaze.

6. Add the oxtail back into the pot, along with any drippings.

7. Close the lid and lock. SEAL the pressure valve.

8. Set to HIGH PRESSURE and cook for 75 minutes.

9. Then QUICK RELEASE.

10. Skim off some of the fat.

11. Whisk the peanut butter and salt into the sauce.

12. Stir in the eggplant and beans.

13. Set to HIGH PRESSURE and cook for 6 minutes.

14. Then QUICK RELEASE.

15. Take out the oxtail and separate the meat from the bones.

16. Add the meat back into the pot along with the fish sauce, if using, and stir.

Nutrition Facts	
(amount per serving)	
Energy (calories)	351
Fat	26.3g
Protein	21.9g
Total Carbohydrates	7.7g
Fiber	2.5g
Net Carbohydrates	5.2g

Macronutrient Breakdown	
Fat	67%
Protein	25%
Carbs	8%

Bolognese Sauce with Zoodles

A hearty meat sauce is such a staple in any menu. Use regular ground beef (70/30) to make it more flavorful and benefit from the healthy fats. If you find it a little too rich, skim off a little of the fat before deglazing the pan or just before serving.

MAKES 4 (1-cup) servings

Spices

2 teaspoons (15.2g) hot paprika

1 tablespoon (3g) dried oregano

2 teaspoons (6g) salt

½ teaspoon (2.5g) Swerve sweetener or erythritol

Meat Sauce

2 tablespoons (30mL) avocado oil

1 medium onion, chopped

2 cloves garlic, minced

1 pound (454g) ground beef

1 stalk celery, diced

¼ cup (60mL) beef or vegetable stock

1 (28oz, 796mL) can crushed tomatoes with liquid

1½ teaspoons (7.5mL) apple cider vinegar

⅓ cup (35g) grated Parmesan cheese, plus more to serve

2 large zucchini, spiralized or grated

red chile flakes, to serve

freshly ground pepper, to serve

1. Mix the spices together and set aside.

PREPARE THE POT

2. Set the pressure cooker to SAUTÉ.

3. When hot, add the olive oil or avocado oil, then sauté the onion until soft, about 1½ minutes.

4. Add the garlic and ground beef and brown the meat.

5. Once brown, stir in the celery.

6. Pour in the stock and stir to deglaze the pot.

7. Mix in the crushed tomatoes, spice mix, apple cider vinegar, and Parmesan cheese.

8. Close the lid and lock. SEAL the pressure valve.

9. Set to HIGH PRESSURE and cook for 3 minutes.

10. Then MANUAL RELEASE PRESSURE after 5 minutes.

11. Mix in the spiralized or grated zucchini.

12. Cover and let sit for 5 minutes.

13. Garnish with red chile flakes, grated Parmesan, and freshly ground pepper to serve, if desired.

VARIATIONS: If you're looking for more than a meat sauce, add in some sliced white mushrooms. Change the flavor up a little and use pork or half pork and half beef. Kick up the seasoning a little and add dried basil, thyme, rosemary, and red chile flakes.

DAIRY-FREE VARIATION: Make it dairy free by omitting the Parmesan cheese.

Nutrition Facts	
(amount per serving)	
Energy (calories)	466
Fat	32g
Protein	27g
Total Carbohydrates	17.5g
Fiber	7.1g
Net Carbohydrates	10.4g

Macronutrient Breakdown	
Fat	62%
Protein	23%
Carbs	14%

Creamy Bolognese Sauce

Sometimes you come home from a long day and you're hungry but not sure what you're going to eat. This was a recipe that came to me by tossing a few things in the pot just to help with hunger. But then my husband raved about it and said I needed to include this dish in the book. So here it is! I'm so happy that he likes what I cook.

MAKES 4 to 5 (1-cup) servings

Spices

2 tablespoons (10g) dried onions

½ teaspoon (0.9g) dried garlic

1 teaspoon (2.3g) paprika

1 tablespoon (2.1g) dried basil

2 teaspoons (12g) sea salt

½ teaspoon (1.4g) ground pepper

Sauce

2 tablespoons (30mL) avocado oil

1 pound (454g) ground beef

1 cup (250mL) beef or vegetable stock

1 (28oz, 796mL) can crushed tomatoes with liquid

1 teaspoon (5mL) Worcestershire sauce

¼ cup (60mL) heavy whipping cream, 33%

¼ cup (25g) grated Parmesan cheese, plus more to serve

2 teaspoons (10mL) cayenne pepper sauce (like Frank's Red Hot)

½ cup (125g) frozen peas and carrots

red chile flakes, to serve

fresh parsley, for garnish, to serve

1. Mix the spices together and set aside.

PREPARE THE POT

2. Set the pressure cooker to SAUTÉ.

3. When hot, add the avocado oil and brown the ground beef.

4. When the meat is about three-quarters cooked, add the spice mix.

5. Once the beef is cooked through, add half of the stock and stir to deglaze the pot.

6. Add the rest of the stock.

7. Stir in the tomatoes and Worcestershire sauce.

8. Close the lid and lock. SEAL the pressure valve.

9. Set to HIGH PRESSURE and cook for 5 minutes.

10. Then MANUAL RELEASE PRESSURE after 1 minute.

11. Stir in the cream and Parmesan cheese.

12. Once incorporated, add the hot sauce.

13. Stir in the peas and carrots.

14. Cover and set the pressure cooker to WARM.

15. Let sit for 2 to 3 minutes before serving with grated Parmesan, red chile flakes, and fresh parsley, if desired.

VARIATION: This sauce uses just a little bit of cream and Parmesan cheese, but could use so much more to make a really nice thick, creamy sauce.

Nutrition Facts	
(amount per serving)	
Energy (calories)	373
Fat	29.7g
Protein	19.6g
Total Carbohydrates	8.1g
Fiber	2.3g
Net Carbohydrates	5.8g

Macronutrient Breakdown	
Fat	71%
Protein	21%
Carbs	8%

Sour Cream Beef

My inspiration for this dish was a beef stroganoff, but it's a little quicker using ground beef rather than thinly sliced.

MAKES 4 (¾-cup) servings

3 slices bacon, cut into 1-inch pieces

¼ cup (34g) chopped onions

1 pound (454g) lean ground beef

1 cup (250mL) beef stock

1 teaspoon (2.3g) paprika

1½ teaspoons (9g) salt

½ teaspoon (1.4g) black pepper

½ cup (121g) sour cream

3 cups (370g) grated or spiralized zucchini, with skin

red chile flakes, to serve

PREPARE THE POT

1. Set the pressure cooker to SAUTÉ.

2. When hot, add the bacon.

3. Move it around to crisp up a little, about 2 to 3 minutes.

4. Add the onions and sauté until just soft, about a minute.

5. Add the ground beef and brown.

6. Once brown, add the beef stock, paprika, salt, and pepper.

7. Close the lid and lock. SEAL the pressure valve.

8. Set to HIGH PRESSURE and cook for 2 minutes.

9. Then QUICK RELEASE.

10. Stir in the sour cream and zucchini.

11. Set the pressure cooker to KEEP WARM.

12. Cover and let sit for 3 to 5 minutes, or until zucchini is at desired tenderness.

13. Garnish with chile flakes and a little freshly ground pepper to serve, if desired.

VARIATIONS: Rather than using ground beef, use beef chunks or stewing beef and cook for 15 to 20 minutes under high pressure, instead of 2 minutes. You could also add in ½ pound of sliced mushrooms, or omit the zucchini and serve the beef and sauce on top of keto-friendly noodles or with spaghetti squash.

DAIRY-FREE VARIATION: Make it dairy free by using coconut milk with cream instead of sour cream.

Nutrition Facts	
(amount per serving)	
Energy (calories)	364
Fat	26g
Protein	27.2g
Total Carbohydrates	4.8g
Fiber	1.1g
Net Carbohydrates	3.7g

Macronutrient Breakdown	
Fat	64%
Protein	30.8%
Carbs	5.2%

Jeff's Favorite Beef Chili

It can be challenging to cook keto-friendly foods that everyone likes, but this is one chili that my husband loves. I normally add a whole cup of black-eyed peas when I'm making it for him, but I've cut it down by half to cut the carbs in half to share it with you.

MAKES 4 to 6 (1-cup) servings

Spices

1 tablespoon (4g) smoked paprika

1 teaspoon (1.5g) red chile flakes

2 teaspoons (12g) salt

1½ teaspoons (3g) ground cumin

1 teaspoon (1g) dried oregano

½ teaspoon (1.4g) coarsely ground black pepper

1 teaspoon (1.8g) cayenne pepper (add another ½ to 1 teaspoon if you like more heat)

Chili

2 tablespoons (30mL) avocado oil or olive oil

1 medium onion, chopped

1 pound (454g) ground beef

2 red, yellow, or orange bell peppers, chopped

2 cloves garlic, minced

1 cup (250mL) beef or vegetable stock

1 (28oz, 796mL) can diced tomatoes with liquid

¼ cup (60mL) sugar-free ketchup

¼ cup (25g) grated Parmesan cheese

1 teaspoon (5mL) Worcestershire sauce

2 teaspoons (10mL) liquid aminos

½ cup (90g) dried black-eyed peas

sliced avocado, to serve

grated cheddar cheese, to serve

chopped cilantro, to serve

guacamole, to serve

chopped green onions, to serve

sour cream, to serve

1. Mix the spices together and set aside.

PREPARE THE POT
2. Set the pressure cooker to SAUTÉ.

3. Once hot, add the avocado oil or olive oil.

4. Add the onion and sauté until translucent, about 1½ minutes.

5. Add the ground beef and brown.

6. Stir in the bell pepper and garlic.

7. Add the stock, tomatoes, ketchup, Parmesan cheese, Worcestershire sauce, and liquid aminos.

8. Stir in the spice mix.

9. Add the dried black-eyed peas.

10. Close the lid and lock. SEAL the pressure valve.

11. Set to HIGH PRESSURE and cook for 60 minutes.

12. Then QUICK RELEASE.

13. Ladle into bowls and serve with your favorite toppings.

VARIATIONS: Rather than use ground beef, use stewing beef cubes for a hearty chili. Try mixing half ground beef, half ground pork. With this chili's bold flavors, venison would be also great. Just add a little more fat to compensate.

DAIRY-FREE VARIATION: Omit the Parmesan cheese.

Nutrition Facts	
(amount per serving)	
Energy (calories)	358
Fat	25.8g
Protein	19.7g
Total Carbohydrates	12.4g
Fiber	3.9g
Net Carbohydrates	8.5g

Macronutrient Breakdown	
Fat	65%
Protein	22%
Carbs	13%

Greek-Inspired Unstuffed Peppers

I've always loved stuffed peppers but have never had the patience to make them and then wait for them to bake. In this recipe, I didn't use green peppers because we don't see eye to eye, but if you like them, feel free to use them.

If riced cauliflower isn't available in the freezer section of your local grocers, it's quite easy to make. Break up the cauliflower into florets and place in a food processor. Pulse until cauliflower bits are about ¼ inch (1cm) size.

MAKES 6 to 7 (¾-cup) servings

Spices

2 teaspoons (2g) dried dill

2 teaspoons (2g) dried oregano

2 teaspoons (2.8g) dried summer savory

2 teaspoons (12g) sea salt

½ teaspoon (1.4g) ground pepper

Ground Beef and Peppers

2 tablespoons (30mL) avocado oil

1 medium onion, chopped

1 pound (454g) ground beef

2 cloves garlic, minced

3 red, yellow, or orange bell peppers, chopped into 1-inch pieces

½ cup (125mL) beef stock or vegetable broth

2½ cups (454g) riced cauliflower (about 1 pound), fresh or frozen

⅔ cup (158g) cubed feta cheese

crumbled feta cheese, to serve

fresh dill sprigs, to serve

lemon wedges, to serve

1. Mix the spices together and set aside.

PREPARE THE POT

2. Set the pressure cooker to SAUTÉ.

3. Once hot, add the avocado oil.

4. Add the onion and sauté until translucent, about 1½ minutes.

5. Add the ground beef and brown.

6. Stir in garlic, then stir in the spice mix.

7. Stir in the bell peppers and beef stock.

8. Close the lid and lock. SEAL the pressure valve.

9. Set to HIGH PRESSURE and cook for 2 minutes.

10. Then QUICK RELEASE.

11. Stir in the riced cauliflower.

12. Close the lid and lock. SEAL the pressure valve.

13. Set to HIGH PRESSURE and cook for 0 minutes to just bring it up to pressure.

14. Then QUICK RELEASE.

15. Mix in cubed feta.

16. Spoon into bowls and serve garnished with crumbled feta, fresh dill, and lemon wedges, if desired.

VARIATIONS: Ground lamb would work especially well with these Greek-inspired seasonings. For an Italian inspiration, use 1 teaspoon dill, replace the summer savory with basil, and add 2 teaspoons thyme to the spice mix. Add 1 to 2 tablespoons tomato paste to the meat mixture and replace the feta with a mixture of Parmesan, Asiago, and Romano cheese.

Nutrition Facts	
(amount per serving)	
Energy (calories)	349
Fat	25.7g
Protein	19.1g
Total Carbohydrates	11g
Fiber	3.5g
Net Carbohydrates	7.5g

Macronutrient Breakdown	
Fat	66%
Protein	22%
Carbs	12%

Cabbage "Roll" Meatloaf

This recipe came about because I had originally planned to make cabbage rolls, but I missed the memo to freeze the cabbage head a few days beforehand to get the leaves nice and soft. I tried popping it in the pressure cooker, but that didn't seem to work for me either. I thought instead I could make a meatloaf out of it!

If riced cauliflower isn't available at your grocery store, it's quite easy to make. Break up the cauliflower into florets and place in a food processor. Pulse until cauliflower bits are about ¼ inch (1cm) size.

MAKES 6 (2½-ounce) servings

Meatloaf Mixture

½ pound (227g) ground beef

½ pound (227g) ground pork

1 teaspoon (1g) dried thyme

1 teaspoon (1g) dried sage

1 teaspoon (1g) dried marjoram

1 teaspoon (3g) salt

½ cup (36g) riced cauliflower, fresh or frozen

1 egg

Sauce Mixture

2 tablespoons (27g) ghee or butter

1 clove garlic, finely minced

1 medium onion, finely chopped

1 (28oz, 796 mL) can diced tomatoes with liquid

1 teaspoon (1g) dried marjoram

1 teaspoon (3g) salt

1 teaspoon (5mL) Worcestershire sauce

¼ to ½ head cabbage, cored and shredded

1. Mix together all the ingredients for the meatloaf in a large bowl. The mixture should be sticky, not crumbly.

2. After mixing well, shape it into a small loaf about 5-inches round and 3-inches tall.

PREPARE THE POT

3. Set the pressure cooker to SAUTÉ, high setting.

4. Once hot, add the ghee or butter.

5. Add the garlic and onion and sauté until soft, about a minute.

6. Add the diced tomatoes with their liquid.

7. Stir in the marjoram, salt, and Worcestershire sauce.

8. Place the meatloaf in the middle of the sauce and make sure it's submerged.

9. Close the lid and lock. SEAL the pressure valve.

10. Set to HIGH PRESSURE and cook for 25 minutes.

11. Then QUICK RELEASE.

12. Check the internal temperature of the meatloaf with an instant-read kitchen thermometer. It should be 160°F when it's done. If not, cook for another 5 to 10 minutes and check again. Once cooked, take out the meatloaf.

13. Mix the shredded cabbage in with the sauce.

14. Close the lid and lock. SEAL the pressure valve.

15. Set to HIGH PRESSURE and cook for 6 minutes.

16. Then MANUAL RELEASE PRESSURE after 1 minute.

17. Slice meatloaf and serve on top of the shredded cabbage with the sauce.

Nutrition Facts	
(amount per serving)	
Energy (calories)	299
Fat	21.3g
Protein	16.4g
Total Carbohydrates	12.3g
Fiber	5.4g
Net Carbohydrates	6.9g

Macronutrient Breakdown	
Fat	64%
Protein	22%
Carbs	16%

CHAPTER 5
Poultry

Chicken Stock

With the pressure cooker, long gone are the days of leaving a pot on the stove overnight to make a flavorful stock, and knowing exactly what's in it by making your own makes chicken stock an excellent staple to have. It's helpful in replenishing electrolytes and nutrients; I drink it when I'm feeling a little off. This makes it perfect for alleviating the keto "flu." Stock also helps layer flavor in so many dishes.

Whenever I pick up rotisserie chicken, I remove most of the meat and immediately freeze the bones. When I've got three carcasses in the freezer, it's time to make stock! If you don't have any handy, check with your local butcher if they've got chicken carcasses or frames. A plus is if they've got wing tips and/or feet too, because that will add some fat and nutritious gelatin to your stock.

MAKES Makes approximately 3 quarts or 12 (1-cup) servings

3 rotisserie chicken carcasses

1 onion, skin on, halved

1 carrot, skin on, halved

2 celery stalks, cut into thirds

1 tablespoon (18g) sea salt

1 teaspoon (1.2g) dried rosemary (optional)

1 teaspoon (1g) dried thyme (optional)

1 large tomato, halved

PREPARE THE POT

1. Add all of the ingredients into the pot.

2. Fill with cool water to 1 inch from the max-fill line.

3. Close the lid and lock. SEAL the pressure valve.

4. Set to HIGH PRESSURE and cook for 75 minutes.

5. Then let the pot NATURAL RELEASE the pressure.

6. Vent steam under the kitchen fan.

7. When cool enough to handle, remove the large pieces of chicken and vegetables. Ladle the stock through a sieve to remove the smaller pieces and spices.

8. Use right away, store in the fridge for 2 to 3 days, or freeze.

TIP: If you'd like to remove some of the fat, rather than skimming it off, refrigerate the stock overnight and then scrape off the fat. For longer storage, add 4 cups of stock to a freezer Ziploc bag, remove the air, and store flat. Fore flavor, especially if the bones are raw, roast the bones in the oven on a foil-lined pan for 350°F for 30 to 45 minutes before making stock.

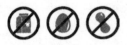

Nutrition facts and macronutrient breakdowns are not included for stocks and broths (see page 26).

Egg Drop Soup

With almost every batch of freshly made chicken broth, I'll make egg drop soup. It's so easy, fast, and nutritious.

MAKES 4 (1-cup) servings

2 eggs, whisked

4 cups (1L) hot fresh chicken stock straight from the pressure cooker

⅛ (0.62mL) teaspoon sesame oil

salt

freshly ground black pepper

chopped green onions, to serve

1. With a fork, whisk the eggs into the hot stock.

2. Add sesame oil, and season to taste with salt and pepper.

3. Ladle into bowls and garnish with green onions.

VARIATIONS: To add a different dimension, use a teaspoon or two of chile oil and liquid aminos. Add some shredded poached chicken for more protein.

Nutrition Facts	
(amount per serving)	
Energy (calories)	103
Fat	8g
Protein	6.3g
Total Carbohydrates	1.2g
Fiber	0g
Net Carbohydrates	1.2g

Macronutrient Breakdown	
Fat	70%
Protein	25%
Carbs	5%

Lemon Chicken Soup

This chicken soup was inspired by the Greek lemon chicken soup avgolemono that I used to have at restaurants, but this version uses riced cauliflower instead of the orzo for more texture and lower carbs. If you don't have any cooked chicken on hand, follow the recipe for Poached Chicken Breasts (page 87) and use the poaching water along with some stock for added flavor.

If riced cauliflower isn't available in the freezer section of your local grocers, it's quite easy to make. Break up the cauliflower into florets and place in a food processor. Pulse until cauliflower bits are about ¼ inch size.

MAKES 5 (1-cup) servings

2 tablespoons (30mL) avocado oil

½ medium onion, chopped fine

¼ cup (35g) small-diced carrot

4 cups (1L) chicken stock

1 bay leaf

1 cup (100g) shredded cooked chicken

2 teaspoons (12g) salt, plus more for seasoning

3 eggs

⅓ cup (80g) lemon juice, from about 2 lemons

¾ cup (72g) riced cauliflower, fresh or frozen

freshly ground pepper

fresh dill, to serve

grated lemon zest, to serve

PREPARE THE POT

1. Set the pressure cooker to SAUTÉ. Once hot, add the avocado oil.

2. Once shimmering, add the onion and carrot, along with a dash of salt. Sauté until the onion is translucent, about 2 minutes.

3. Add the stock, bay leaf, chicken, and salt.

4. Close the lid and lock. SEAL the pressure valve.

5. Set to HIGH PRESSURE and cook for 5 minutes.

6. Then QUICK RELEASE.

7. While the stock is cooking, whisk eggs well then mix in the lemon juice.

8. When the cooking time is complete, ladle about 1 cup of only the hot liquid into a bowl and set aside.

9. Add the riced cauliflower to the rest of the soup in the pressure cooker and let sit.

10. While whisking quickly, slowly add 1 tablespoon at a time of the reserved hot broth to the egg lemon mixture. This prevents curdling. The egg-broth mixture should be about the same temperature as the soup in the pressure cooker.

11. While stirring, slowly add the egg mixture back into the pressure cooker.

12. Let sit for about a minute, and season with salt and pepper to taste.

13. Serve garnished with fresh dill and grated lemon zest, if desired.

VARIATIONS: If you want to change the flavors a little, consider adding thyme, rosemary, or dill in place or addition to the bay leaf. Looking to add a little more? Add some chopped celery or leeks to sweeten the soup up a little.

Nutrition Facts	
(amount per serving)	
Energy (calories)	132
Fat	9.3g
Protein	8.3g
Total Carbohydrates	3.8g
Fiber	0.8g
Net Carbohydrates	3g

Macronutrient Breakdown	
Fat	62%
Protein	26%
Carbs	11%

Creamy Tarragon, Sage, and Mushroom Chicken Soup

Tarragon is such an underutilized herb. It goes great with fish and beautifully with chicken, and it makes this soup stand out. For an extra treat, try serving it with cooked crumbled bacon on top.

MAKES 8 (¾-cup) servings

Spices

¼ teaspoon (0.7g) ground pepper

1 tablespoon (1g) dried tarragon

1 teaspoon (0.8g) dried marjoram

2 sprigs fresh sage

2 teaspoons (12g) sea salt

½ teaspoon (1.2g) ground mustard

Soup

2 strips bacon, cut into ½-inch pieces

6 boneless, skinless chicken breasts (3½ pounds, 1.6kg)

½ medium onion, chopped

6 cups (1.5L) chicken stock

1 pound (454g)white mushrooms, sliced

½ brick (4oz, 125g) cream cheese, cut into 4

¼ cup (60mL) heavy cream, 33%

1. Mix the spices together, then set aside.

PREPARE THE POT

2. Set the pressure cooker to SAUTÉ.

3. Once hot, add the bacon. Stir the bacon around every 30 seconds.

4. Remove the bacon when it is just getting crisp, about 4 minutes.

5. Brown the chicken breasts, about 2 minutes each side. Remove and set aside.

6. Add the onion and sauté until soft and translucent, about a minute.

7. Pour in the chicken stock and stir to deglaze the pot. Then mix in spices.

8. Return the bacon and chicken to the pot along with any drippings.

9. Close the lid and lock. SEAL the pressure valve.

10. Set to HIGH PRESSURE and cook for 7 minutes.

11. Then QUICK RELEASE.

12. Remove the chicken, shred with two forks, and set aside.

13. Set the pressure cooker to SAUTÉ.

14. Add the mushrooms, then whisk in the cream cheese and cream.

15. Add chicken back in along with any drippings.

16. Close the lid and lock. SEAL the pressure valve.

17. Set to HIGH PRESSURE and cook for 7 minutes.

18. Then QUICK RELEASE.

19. Remove the sage before serving.

VARIATION: Omit the mustard and replace the tarragon with dill and this soup takes on a whole different flavor.

Nutrition Facts	
(amount per serving)	
Energy (calories)	327
Fat	20.6g
Protein	31.1g
Total Carbohydrates	3.9g
Fiber	1g
Net Carbohydrates	2.9g

Macronutrient Breakdown	
Fat	56%
Protein	38%
Carbs	5.7%

Vegetable Chicken Soup

I have never made minestrone soup before, but my husband loves it. He says this soup reminds him of it.

MAKES 6 (1-cup) servings

Spices

2 teaspoons (1.4g) dried basil

1 tablespoon (1.8g) fresh sage

1 tablespoon (2.4g) fresh thyme

1 tablespoon (3.3g) fresh dill

1 tablespoon (18g) sea salt

½ teaspoon (1.4g) freshly ground pepper

1 bay leaf

Soup

2 tablespoons (30mL) avocado oil

4 chicken thighs and 4 chicken drumsticks, bone-in, skin-on, about 2¾ pounds (1.3kg)

1 medium onion, chopped

2 cloves garlic, minced

1 cup (40g) medium-diced celery (about 1 stalk)

1 cup (100g) medium-diced carrot

2 cups (500mL) chicken stock

1 (28oz, 798mL) can diced tomatoes with liquid

1 tablespoon (16g) tomato paste

1 cup (150g) medium-diced zucchini

1 cup (80g) sliced bok choy

¼ cup (30g) grated Parmesan cheese

salt

freshly ground pepper

fresh dill, to serve

1. Mix together the herbs and spices and set aside.

PREPARE THE POT

2. Set the pressure cooker to SAUTÉ, high setting.

3. Once hot, add the avocado oil.

4. Sprinkle a little salt and pepper on the chicken.

5. Brown both sides of the chicken in batches, about 2 to 3 minutes per side. Remove and set aside.

6. Add the onion, garlic, celery, and carrot, and sauté for 2 to 3 minutes, until the onion softens.

7. Pour in the stock and stir to deglaze the pot.

8. Stir in the tomatoes, then whisk in the tomato paste.

9. Stir in the spices and return the chicken to pot along with any drippings.

10. Close the lid and lock. SEAL the pressure valve.

11. Set to HIGH PRESSURE and cook for 15 minutes.

12. Then QUICK RELEASE.

13. Remove the chicken, shred with two forks, and set aside.

14. Add the chicken back to the pot, along with any juices.

15. Add the zucchini, bok choy, and Parmesan cheese.

16. Close the lid and lock. SEAL the pressure valve.

17. Set to HIGH PRESSURE and cook for 2 minutes.

18. Then QUICK RELEASE.

19. Ladle into bowls and garnish with fresh dill to serve.

DAIRY-FREE VARIATION: Make it dairy free by omitting the Parmesan cheese and adding ½ teaspoon Worcestershire sauce.

VEGETARIAN VARIATION: Make it vegetarian by omitting the chicken and replacing the chicken stock with vegetable stock.

VEGAN VARIATION: Make it vegan by omitting the chicken, replacing the chicken stock with vegetable stock, and omitting the Parmesan cheese.

Nutrition Facts	
(amount per serving)	
Energy (calories)	376
Fat	24.8g
Protein	27.2g
Total Carbohydrates	12.1g
Fiber	4.8g
Net Carbohydrates	7.3g

Macronutrient Breakdown	
Fat	59%
Protein	29%
Carbs	12%

Roasted Whole Chicken

There's nothing like having a roasted chicken. Starting it off in the pressure cooker ensures a wonderfully juicy bird, and finishing it in the oven gives it that crispy skin that everyone loves.

MAKES 4 to 6 (4-ounce) servings

Marinade

2 tablespoons (30mL) avocado oil

2 tablespoons (30mL) cider vinegar

1 tablespoons (18g) salt

1 teaspoon (2.8g) freshly ground black pepper

1 teaspoon (5g) Dijon mustard

2 cloves garlic, crushed

1 tablespoon (6.8g) hot paprika

1 tablespoon (3g) dried thyme

1 tablespoon (3g) dried oregano

1 tablespoon (2.1g) dried basil

½ teaspoon (1.8g) cayenne pepper

Chicken

1 whole chicken, about 5 pounds (2kg)

½ cup (125mL) chicken stock

1 medium lemon

2 tablespoons (30mL) olive oil

1. Mix all the marinade ingredients in a large Ziploc bag that's big enough to fit the whole chicken.

2. Place the chicken in the bag with the marinade and seal. Spread the marinade around the chicken.

3. Let marinate for 4 to 24 hours in the fridge.

4. When ready to cook, take the chicken out of the fridge.

PREPARE THE POT

5. Add the chicken stock to the pot and put it in the flat steamer rack.

6. Poke holes all over the lemon with a fork and insert the lemon in the chicken cavity.

7. Place the chicken on top of the steamer rack. Pour the marinade from the bag on top of the chicken.

8. Close the lid and lock. SEAL the pressure valve.

9. Set to HIGH PRESSURE and cook for 17 minutes.

10. Then QUICK RELEASE.

11. Transfer the chicken to the pan and let it rest for 10 minutes.

12. In the meantime, preheat the oven to 425°F.

13. Pat the chicken dry and baste with olive oil.

14. Put the chicken in oven for 30 minutes.

15. If the skin is not crispy, broil the chicken on high for 5 minutes then flip and broil the underside for 5 minutes.

16. Allow to rest for 10 minutes.

17. Stir together the sauce from the pressure cooker and the drippings from the pan.

18. Carve the chicken and serve with the sauce.

VARIATION: Rather than cooking one chicken, try using two Cornish game hens.

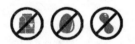

Nutrition Facts	
(amount per serving)	
Energy (calories)	252
Fat	15g
Protein	27g
Total Carbohydrates	0g
Fiber	0g
Net Carbohydrates	0g

Macronutrient Breakdown	
Fat	54%
Protein	43%
Carbs	0%

Hainanese Chicken

I don't know what it is about Hainanese chicken that I like so much. The meat is juicy and succulent with subtle notes of the ginger and onion. The skin has a texture that may be challenging for some, but just take it off and save it for chicken skin chips (just pop them under the broiler!). Usually Hainanese chicken is served with rice, but it's also great on its own with just a little dipping sauce. A big thanks to Pedro and Ale for trying this out!

MAKES 4 to 6 (4-ounce) servings

Chicken

1 whole chicken, about 5 pounds (2kg)

coarse salt

1 tablespoon (15mL) sesame oil

4 inches (10.2cm) fresh ginger, peeled, cut into 1-inch sections and smashed

1 bunch spring onions

Dipping Sauce

½ cup (125mL) cooking liquid from the pressure cooker

2 tablespoons (30mL) liquid aminos

½ teaspoon (2.5g) sambal oelek chile paste

1. To prepare the chicken, clean it by rubbing coarse salt all over the skin without breaking it. Rinse and pat dry.

2. Season inside and outside the chicken with salt and sesame oil.

3. Stuff ginger and spring onions inside the bird.

PREPARE THE POT

4. Add 2 cups of water to the pot and put it in the flat steamer rack.

5. Place the chicken on the rack.

6. Close the lid and lock. SEAL the pressure valve.

7. Set to HIGH PRESSURE and cook for 17 minutes.

8. Then QUICK RELEASE.

9. Take out the chicken and let it rest on a platter for 10 minutes.

10. Whisk the ingredients together for the dipping sauce.

11. Carve the chicken and serve with the sauce.

VARIATION: In addition to the dipping sauce, for those that want a more bold flavor, try mixing a little sriracha into the dipping sauce or just serving it as a dipping sauce on its own.

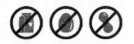

Nutrition Facts	
(amount per serving)	
Energy (calories)	202
Fat	7.65g
Protein	31g
Total Carbohydrates	0g
Fiber	0g
Net Carbohydrates	0g

Macronutrient Breakdown	
Fat	34%
Protein	62%
Carbs	0%

Rustic Italian Chicken

I love using capers, Kalamata olives, and sun-dried tomatoes together, and they work really well in this dish. It's one that can be a little salty, which is great to help keep up electrolytes, but you may want to hold off on the salt and season to taste.

MAKES 4 (4½-ounce) servings, about 1½ thighs each

2 tablespoons (30mL) avocado oil

2 pounds (900g) chicken thighs, skin-on, bone-in

½ cup (55g) diced onion

2 garlic cloves, minced

6 Roma tomatoes, chopped

⅓ cup (80mL) chicken stock

2 sun-dried tomato halves, chopped

2 tablespoons (19g) capers, drained

⅓ cup (60g) pitted Kalamata olives

3 sprigs fresh oregano

1 teaspoon (6g) salt

lemon wedges, to serve

PREPARE THE POT

1. Set the pressure cooker to SAUTÉ, higher setting.

2. When hot, add the avocado oil.

3. Brown the chicken on both sides in batches, about 2 to 3 minutes per side, taking care not to overcrowd the pan. Remove and set aside.

4. Add the chopped onion and garlic, and sauté for 30 seconds.

5. When fragrant, add in one-third of the chopped tomatoes, and stir to break them down to a mush.

6. Pour in the chicken stock and stir to deglaze the pot.

7. Stir in the sun-dried tomato, capers, olives, oregano, salt.

8. Add the chicken back in, along with any drippings.

9. Close the lid and lock. SEAL the pressure valve.

10. Set to HIGH PRESSURE and cook for 10 minutes.

11. Then QUICK RELEASE.

12. Serve the chicken thighs with lemon wedges.

VARIATION: Use chicken breasts or pork loin chops instead, and cook for 6 minutes under high pressure. Once cooked, shred the chicken and serve on top of Cauliflower Mash (page 186).

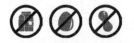

Nutrition Facts	
(amount per serving)	
Energy (calories)	551
Fat	52.9g
Protein	12.7g
Total Carbohydrates	7.1g
Fiber	2g
Net Carbohydrates	5.1g

Macronutrient Breakdown	
Fat	86%
Protein	9%
Carbs	5%

Chicken Cacciatore

Cacciatore, known as hunter's stew, uses many bold flavors to season the wild catch of the day. I've used chicken quarters and their dark meat to help bring out the flavors, but don't let that stop you from using chicken breasts either. Pair this dish with cauliflower rice or a plain Cauliflower Mash (page 186) so the flavors don't compete.

MAKES 6 (4½-ounce) servings

2 tablespoons (30mL) avocado oil

4 chicken thighs and 4 chicken drumsticks, bone-in, skin-on, about 3 pounds (1.3kg)

1 medium onion, chopped

1 medium red bell pepper, chopped

3 cloves garlic, minced

1 cup (250mL) chicken or vegetable stock

2 tablespoons (32g) tomato paste

1 (28-ounce, 796mL) can diced tomatoes with liquid

¼ cup (60mL) apple cider vinegar

3 tablespoons (25g) capers, drained

1 tablespoon (2g) dried basil

2 teaspoons (2g) dried oregano

1 teaspoon (2g) red chile flakes

2 teaspoons (10mL) Worcestershire sauce

salt

freshly ground black pepper

PREPARE THE POT

1. Set the pressure cooker to SAUTÉ, higher setting.

2. Once hot, add the avocado oil.

3. Sprinkle salt and pepper on chicken.

4. Brown both sides of the chicken in batches, about 2 to 3 minutes per side. Remove and set aside.

5. Add the onion and red bell pepper, and sauté for 2 to 3 minutes, until the onion softens.

6. Sprinkle in salt and pepper to taste.

7. Add the garlic and stir for 30 seconds.

8. Pour in the stock and stir to deglaze the pot.

9. Whisk in the tomato paste.

10. Stir in the tomatoes, vinegar, capers, basil, oregano, red chile flakes, and Worcestershire sauce.

11. Return the chicken and any drippings back to the pot.

12. Close the lid and lock. SEAL the pressure valve.

13. Set to HIGH PRESSURE and cook for 14 minutes.

14. Then QUICK RELEASE.

15. From two thighs, shred the meat with skin and discard the bone. Stir the shredded meat into the sauce.

16. Serve a drumstrick or thigh with a ladle of sauce.

VARIATIONS: As this is a "hunter's stew," try using pork, rabbit, venison, or even turkey instead of chicken.

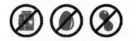

Nutrition Facts	
(amount per serving)	
Energy (calories)	434
Fat	29.6g
Protein	33.6g
Total Carbohydrates	6.9g
Fiber	1.9g
Net Carbohydrates	5g

Macronutrient Breakdown	
Fat	62.2%
Protein	31.4%
Carbs	6.4%

Chicken Mushroom Alfredo Zoodles

I just love full meals that come together in one pot and that are tasty and nutritious in less than an hour of cooking after a long day at work. This chicken mushroom Alfredo is comfort food.

MAKES 4 (4-ounce) servings

2 tablespoons (27g) ghee, butter, or avocado oil

2 fresh boneless, skinless chicken breasts, about 1¼ pounds (544g)

½ medium onion, diced

1 clove garlic, minced

½ cup (125mL) chicken stock

6 white mushrooms, sliced

2 teaspoons (12g) salt

½ cup (125mL) heavy cream, 33%

¼ cup (25g) grated Parmesan cheese, plus more to serve

1 medium zucchini, spiralized or grated

red chile flakes, to serve

freshly ground pepper, to serve

fresh parsley, to serve

PREPARE THE POT

1. Set the pressure cooker to SAUTÉ, higher setting.

2. Once hot, melt the ghee or butter, or add the avocado oil.

3. Brown the chicken breasts, about 2 minutes each side, then set aside.

4. Add the onion and garlic, and sauté until the onion is soft, about 1 minute.

5. Pour in the stock and stir to deglaze the pot.

6. Add the chicken breasts back in along with any juices.

7. Set to HIGH PRESSURE and cook for 5 minutes.

8. Then QUICK RELEASE.

9. Remove the chicken and let rest.

10. Set the pressure cooker to SAUTÉ.

11. Add the mushrooms and salt, and sauté for about 1 minute.

12. Whisk in the cream, then the Parmesan cheese.

13. Add the zucchini.

14. Cut up the chicken into cubes and return to the pot, along with any liquid.

15. Set the pressure cooker to WARM.

16. Let heat through for 1 to 3 minutes, or until the zoodles are a desired tenderness.

17. Serve with grated Parmesan, red chile flakes, pepper, and parsley, if desired.

VARIATIONS: Use ground turkey or chicken. Add 2 to 3 tablespoons of cream cheese to boost fats and to make it creamier. Leave out the zucchini and use the sauce with a low-carb black bean noodle.

Nutrition Facts	
(amount per serving)	
Energy (calories)	455
Fat	32.8g
Protein	33.7g
Total Carbohydrates	6.6g
Fiber	1.5g
Net Carbohydrates	5.1g

Macronutrient Breakdown	
Fat	65%
Protein	30%
Carbs	6%

Chicken with Creamy Tomato Sauce

This hearty meal is one of those simple dishes for a cold day. The cream gives the dish body. Feel free to add a little more to make it even richer!

MAKES 4 (1½-cup) servings

¼ cup (60mL) chicken stock or water

2 cups (500mL) tomato sauce

2 boneless, skinless chicken breasts, about 1¼ pounds (544g), frozen

2 tablespoons (30mL) heavy cream, 33%

salt

chopped cilantro, to serve

grated Parmesan cheese, to serve

PREPARE THE POT

1. Add the chicken stock or water to the pressure cooker.

2. Stir in the tomato sauce.

3. Add the chicken, and spoon some sauce over the top to cover.

4. Close the lid and lock. SEAL the pressure valve.

5. Set to HIGH PRESSURE and cook for 8 to 9 minutes.

6. Then QUICK RELEASE.

7. Remove the chicken, shred with two forks, and set aside.

8. Stir the cream into the sauce.

9. Mix the chicken along with any liquid back into the sauce.

10. Season with salt to taste.

11. Serve with cilantro and Parmesan cheese, if desired.

VARIATIONS: For more added fat, use chicken thighs with skin. Use spices such as garlic, rosemary, and basil to boost this dish's flavor. Try it with pork chops or pork loin steaks.

Nutrition Facts	
(amount per serving)	
Energy (calories)	290
Fat	15.7g
Protein	30g
Total Carbohydrates	6.8g
Fiber	1.9g
Net Carbohydrates	4.9g

Macronutrient Breakdown	
Fat	49%
Protein	41%
Carbs	9%

Poached Chicken Breasts

This method is good for when you've forgotten to let chicken thaw, because it's quick, easy, and hands off. Some recipes like the Quick and Easy Butter Chicken (page 99) recipe become much easier when you have precooked chicken on hand.

Making chicken salad or meal prepping couldn't be any easier with these simple chicken breasts. The trick is just to make sure that no matter how many breasts you're cooking, all are submerged under the poaching liquid. Check the internal temperature for doneness, 165°F (74°C), using an instant-read kitchen thermometer. When you're done cooking, drink the poaching liquid or save it in the fridge and use it as broth.

MAKES 2 (5-ounce) servings, about ½ chicken breast each

1 cup (250mL) chicken stock	½ teaspoon (3g) salt
1 cup (250mL) water	pinch freshly ground pepper
½ teaspoon (0.5g) thyme, dried	1 chicken breast, (9oz, 272g), frozen

PREPARE THE POT

1. Add the stock and water to the pot.

2. Add the thyme, salt, and pepper to the liquid.

3. Place the chicken in the poaching liquid. Make sure it is submerged. If not, add a little more water.

4. Close the lid and lock. SEAL the pressure valve.

5. Set to HIGH PRESSURE and cook for 12 minutes.

6. Then QUICK RELEASE.

7. Remove the chicken and shred with two forks. Or let rest for a minute before slicing.

SERVING SUGGESTIONS:

Use in chicken salad, chicken Caesar salad, or for Quick and Easy Butter Chicken (page 99).

Heat up some chicken stock along with a little celery and carrot, and drop some chicken in for a fast chicken soup.

Shred chicken and mix in some salsa, sour cream, and guacamole. Serve in a lettuce cup or a wrap.

Shred chicken and toss with a little liquid aminos, sriracha, a drop of sesame oil, and some chopped green onions. Serve over low-carb noodles or shirataki noodles.

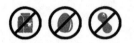

Nutrition Facts	
(amount per serving)	
Energy (calories)	163
Fat	3.6g
Protein	30.6g
Total Carbohydrates	0g
Fiber	0g
Net Carbohydrates	0g

Macronutrient Breakdown	
Fat	19.7%
Protein	5%
Carbs	0%

Chile Chicken and Eggs

This recipe came about after a long day at work with no real dinner plan, and I was pretty happy with the way it turned out. When the egg on top is broken, the yolk adds more creaminess and body to an already flavorful sauce.

MAKES 4 (5-ounce) servings

2 tablespoons (25g) ghee, butter, or avocado oil

½ medium onion, diced

1½ slices bacon, cut into 1-inch pieces

½ cup (125mL) chicken stock

1 cup (180g) chopped tomato (about 1 large tomato)

¼ cup (62g) sugar-free ketchup

1 tablespoon (8g) chile powder

2 teaspoons (12g) salt

2 boneless, skinless chicken breasts, about 1¼ pounds (544g), fresh or frozen

¼ cup (60mL) sour cream, plus more to serve

4 eggs

PREPARE THE POT

1. Set the pressure cooker to SAUTÉ.

2. When hot, add the ghee or butter or oil.

3. Add the onion and sauté until soft, about a minute.

4. Add the bacon and cook for 1 to 2 minutes until warmed up but not crisp.

5. Pour in the stock and stir to deglaze the pot.

6. Add the tomato, ketchup, chile powder, and salt. Stir to combine.

7. Add the chicken breasts. Make sure they're submerged and touching the bottom of the pan.

8. Close the lid and lock. SEAL the pressure valve.

9. If using fresh chicken, set to HIGH PRESSURE and cook for 5 to 6 minutes; if using frozen chicken, set to HIGH PRESSURE and cook for 10 to 12 minutes.

10. Then QUICK RELEASE.

11. Check for doneness. Cook for an additional 2 to 3 minutes, if necessary.

12. Remove the chicken, shred it with two forks, and return it to the pot.

13. Stir in the sour cream.

14. Draw an "X" on the surface of the sauce with a spoon to divide it into 4 sections.

15. Crack 1 egg into a small bowl or glass.

16. Carefully pour the egg into one of the 4 sections without piercing the yolk. Repeat with the remaining eggs. Do *not* mix.

17. Close the lid and lock. SEAL the pressure valve.

18. Set to HIGH PRESSURE and cook for 0 minutes just to bring it up to pressure *or* set to LOW PRESSURE and cook for 4 minutes.

19. Then QUICK RELEASE.

20. To serve, carefully scoop a generous portion of the chicken chile with the egg on top into a bowl. Top with sour cream, if desired.

VARIATION: To make it spicier, add ½ teaspoon of cayenne pepper.

DAIRY-FREE VARIATION: Make it dairy free by omitting the sour cream and using avocado oil.

Nutrition Facts	
(amount per serving)	
Energy (calories)	458
Fat	30.5g
Protein	36.4g
Total Carbohydrates	9.2g
Fiber	1.5g
Net Carbohydrates	7.7g

Macronutrient Breakdown	
Fat	60%
Protein	32%
Carbs	8%

Chicken Tinga (Chipotle Tomato Chicken)

I've always been drawn to canned chipotle chiles with adobo sauce. I know they're just smoked jalapeños, but they're packed with that wonderful smoky flavor, and the heat is a bonus! This recipe is just an excuse to use a can. Try serving this in a low-carb wrap, lettuce wrap, or even a cheese taco shell.

MAKES 4 to 5 (6-ounce) servings

2 tablespoons (30mL) avocado oil

½ medium onion, sliced

1 clove garlic, minced

1 (28oz, 796mL) can diced tomatoes

1 (7oz, 199g) can chipotle chiles with adobo sauce, chopped

4 boneless, skinless chicken breasts, about 2 pounds (880g), fresh or frozen

salt

freshly ground pepper

chopped cilantro, to serve

guacamole, to serve

lime wedges, to serve

shredded cheddar cheese, to serve

sour cream, to serve

PREPARE THE POT

1. Set the pressure cooker to SAUTÉ.

2. When hot, add the avocado oil.

3. Add the onion and sauté until softened, about a minute.

4. Add the garlic, the tomatoes, including half their liquid, and the chopped chipotles with sauce, and season with salt and pepper. Stir to combine.

5. Add the chicken breasts. Make sure they're not overlapping and that they're submerged in the sauce.

6. Close the lid and lock. SEAL the pressure valve.

7. If using fresh chicken, set to HIGH PRESSURE and cook for 5 to 6 minutes; if using frozen chicken, set to HIGH PRESSURE and cook for 12 minutes.

8. Then QUICK RELEASE.

9. Check for doneness, especially if starting with frozen chicken. Cook for an additional 2 minutes if necessary.

10. Keep whole or slice or shred, as desired.

11. Serve with a generous portion of sauce, along with cilantro, guacamole, lime wedges, cheese, and sour cream, if desired.

VARIATIONS: Need to bump up some fats? Try adding bacon, butter, cream, or even medium-chain triglyceride (MCT) oil after cooking! Another way to add good fat is to use chicken thighs or drumsticks with skin.

DAIRY-FREE VARIATION: Omit the cheese and sour cream or replace the cheddar cheese and dairy sour cream with vegan cheese and a vegan sour cream.

Nutrition Facts	
(amount per serving)	
Energy (calories)	374
Fat	22g
Protein	37.6g
Total Carbohydrates	5.1g
Fiber	1.6g
Net Carbohydrates	3.5g

Macronutrient Breakdown	
Fat	53%
Protein	40%
Carbs	5%

Chicken Verde

When I heard how easy it is to make salsa verde, I just had to try it out myself. Sure enough, it is pretty easy since the food processor does the heavy lifting. I like to make a lot and keep some in the fridge. There's nothing like fresh salsa verde, and then to use that on top of chicken in the pressure cooker is simply delicious!

MAKES 12 (5-ounce) servings

Salsa Verde

2 poblano chiles, halved and seeded

3 jalapeños, halved and seeded

1 medium onion, halved

2 cloves garlic

5 tomatillos, halved and husked

2 teaspoons (2.1g) ground cumin

2 teaspoons (2g) dried oregano

zest and juice of 1 lime

2 teaspoons (12g) salt

1 jalapeño, halved (optional)

½ bunch cilantro, stems removed (optional)

Chicken

1 cup (250mL) chicken stock

6 chicken breasts, about 3¾ pounds (1.6kg), fresh or frozen

chopped cilantro, to serve

lime wedges, to serve

sour cream, to serve

shredded cheddar cheese, to serve

1. Line a cookie sheet with foil and preheat the oven's broiler.

2. Place the salsa verde ingredients on the cookie sheet.

3. Place the pan under the broiler for about 15 minutes, then turn over and roast for about another 10, until the vegetables are roasted and slightly charred.

4. Trim the onion ends and discard. Place the onions in a food processor with the chiles, garlic, tomatillos, cumin, oregano, lime juice and zest, salt, cilantro, and jalapeño, if desired for extra heat. Pulse until pureed and no large chunks remain, approximately 12 pulses depending on the size of your processor.

PREPARE THE POT

5. Add the chicken stock to the pressure cooker.

6. Place the chicken in the pot and spread the fresh salsa verde on top. Make sure the chicken is completely covered.

7. Close the lid and lock. SEAL the pressure valve.

8. Set to HIGH PRESSURE and cook for 5 to 6 minutes for fresh chicken, or 12 to 15 minutes for frozen.

9. Then MANUAL RELEASE PRESSURE after 2 to 3 minutes.

10. Remove the chicken, shred it with two forks, and add it back into the sauce.

11. Serve with a generous dollop of sour cream and chedddar cheese to bump up some fats, along with the lime juice and cilantro, if desired.

VARIATIONS: Using a darker meat such as chicken thighs or drumsticks would add a little more flavor, especially with the skin on. A nice white fish would rock this for fish tacos, just cut the cook time in half.

Nutrition Facts (amount per serving)	
Energy (calories)	172
Fat	8.3g
Protein	19.1g
Total Carbohydrates	5.1g
Fiber	1.1g
Net Carbohydrates	4g

Macronutrient Breakdown	
Fat	43%
Protein	44%
Carbs	11%

Chicken with Bacon, Chorizo, and Ancho Chile

There's so much goodness going on in this dish, you'll want to lick the bowl. Serving this with something like cauliflower rice for soaking up the sauce would be perfect.

MAKES 8 (½-cup) servings

Spices

½ teaspoon (1.4g) freshly ground pepper

½ teaspoon (1.1g) red chile flakes

½ teaspoon (1g) ground cumin

½ teaspoon (1.1g) paprika

¼ teaspoon (0.8g) ground cinnamon

2 teaspoons (12g) sea salt

2 teaspoons (7g) ancho chile powder

Chicken

4 strips bacon, cut into ½-inch pieces

6 bone-in, skin-on chicken thighs, about 2 pounds (900g)

½ medium onion, chopped

2 links chorizo sausage, casing removed

1 cup (250mL) chicken stock

½ cup (125g) sugar-free ketchup

1. Mix the spices together and set aside.

PREPARE THE POT

2. Set the cooker to SAUTÉ, higher setting.

3. Once hot, add the bacon and stir every 30 seconds.

4. Remove the bacon when it is just getting crisp, about 4 to 5 minutes.

5. Brown the chicken thighs, about 2 minutes on each side, then remove and set aside.

6. Carefully remove any excess bacon fat, leaving about 2 tablespoons in the pot.

7. Add the onion and sauté until soft and translucent, about a minute.

8. Add in the chorizo sausage and brown.

9. Pour in the stock and stir to deglaze the pot.

10. Stir in the spices and ketchup.

11. Return the bacon and chicken to the pot along with any drippings.

12. Close the lid and lock. SEAL the pressure valve.

13. Set to HIGH PRESSURE and cook for 10 minutes.

14. Then MANUAL RELEASE PRESSURE after 10 minutes.

15. Remove the bones from the chicken thighs and return the meat to the pot. Mix.

16. Ladle into bowls on top of cauliflower rice if desired.

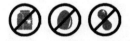

Nutrition Facts	
(amount per serving)	
Energy (calories)	381
Fat	29g
Protein	24.3g
Total Carbohydrates	2.9g
Fiber	1.4g
Net Carbohydrates	1.5g

Macronutrient Breakdown	
Fat	71%
Protein	24.3%
Carbs	2.2%

Buffalo Wings

This is a quick, simple recipe. There's nothing too complex, and it satisfies cravings for wings on a weeknight. Serve with celery sticks or a leafy green salad and your favorite dipping sauce (even Caesar dressing works in a pinch!). Hint: The leftover steam water in the pot makes a couple of cups of chicken broth you can pop in the fridge and use later.

MAKES 3 to 4 servings, 6 wings each

Spices

2 teaspoons (4.6g) paprika

2 teaspoons (12g) salt

½ teaspoon (0.5g) dried oregano, dried

½ teaspoon (1.4g) coarsely ground black pepper

Buffalo Wings

2¼ pounds (1kg) chicken wings, split and tips removed (about 24 pieces), patted dry

¼ cup (125mL) cayenne pepper sauce (like Frank's Red Hot)

¼ cup (½ stick, 56g) salted butter, melted

½ teaspoon (0.9g) garlic powder

blue cheese or ranch dressing, to serve

1. Mix the spices together. Sprinkle over the chicken wings and toss to coat.

PREPARE THE POT

2. Add 1½ cups cool water to the pot.

3. Place a vegetable steamer basket in the pot.

4. Arrange the wings in the basket. Try to keep them in a single layer.

5. Close the lid and lock. SEAL the pressure valve.

6. Set to HIGH PRESSURE and cook for 12 minutes.

7. Then QUICK RELEASE.

8. While wings are cooking, whisk together the cayenne pepper sauce, melted butter, and garlic powder.

9. When the wings are done, toss them in the sauce.

10. Serve with blue cheese or ranch dressing for dipping.

VARIATIONS: I often have some sauce on hand from Quick and Easy Butter Chicken (page 99). Warming up a cup to pour over the wings is easy and tasty!

Nutrition Facts	
(amount per serving)	
Energy (calories)	410
Fat	32.5g
Protein	28.1g
Total Carbohydrates	1.8g
Fiber	0.7g
Net Carbohydrates	1.1g

Macronutrient Breakdown	
Fat	71%
Protein	27%
Carbs	2%

Quick and Easy Butter Chicken

This recipe becomes even easier if you use a rotisserie chicken for a quick midweek meal. Serve with cauliflower rice.

MAKES 6 (4-ounce) servings

2 tablespoons (27g) ghee, butter, or avocado oil

1⅛ teaspoons (6.8g) salt

½ teaspoon (1.4g) freshly ground black pepper

1½ pounds (680g) boneless, skinless chicken breasts, cut into 1-inch cubes (about 4 to 5 breasts)

1 medium onion, diced

2 cloves garlic, minced

1½ teaspoons (6g) grated fresh ginger

2 teaspoons (6g) garam masala

1½ teaspoons (3.5g) paprika

3 green cardamom pods (optional)

1 black cardamom pod (optional)

½ teaspoons (0.9g) cayenne pepper (optional)

1 small green chile pepper, chopped (add 1 more for extra heat)

½ cup (125mL) chicken stock

1 cup (250mL) tomato sauce or crushed tomatoes

1 tablespoon (16g) tomato paste

1 cup (250mL) heavy cream, 33%

PREPARE THE POT

1. Set the pressure cooker to SAUTÉ.

2. Once hot, melt the ghee or butter, or add the avocado oil.

3. Sprinkle the salt and pepper on the chicken.

4. Add the chicken and sauté it until all sides are just cooked, about 4 to 5 minutes. Remove and set aside.

5. Add the onion, garlic, and ginger, and sauté until the onion is soft, about a minute.

6. Add the garam masala, paprika, cardamom pods and cayenne, if using, and the green chile. Stir to toast and activate the spices, about 1 to 2 minutes.

7. Pour in the stock and stir to deglaze the pot.

8. Add the tomato sauce and whisk in the tomato paste.

9. Return the chicken and any juices back to the pan.

10. Close the lid and lock. SEAL the pressure valve.

11. Set to HIGH PRESSURE and cook for 3 to 4 minutes.

12. Then QUICK RELEASE.

13. Set the pressure cooker to SAUTÉ.

14. Whisk in the cream. Continue stirring until the cream has warmed through and is just starting to bubble, about 1 to 2 minutes.

15. Remove the green chile pepper and cardamom pods, if they were added.

VARIATION: Make the sauce without the chicken and use it as a cream sauce for other dishes.

DAIRY-FREE VARIATION: Make it dairy free by replacing the ghee or butter with coconut oil and using coconut milk instead of cream.

Nutrition Facts	
(amount per serving)	
Energy (calories)	410
Fat	30.9g
Protein	25.8g
Total Carbohydrates	8.3g
Fiber	1.7g
Net Carbohydrates	6.6g

Macronutrient Breakdown	
Fat	67%
Protein	25%
Carbs	8%

Opor Ayam (Indonesian Coconut Chicken)

A friend had mentioned this dish to me while I was on the hunt for new recipes. It sounded interesting but I really wasn't sure how it would turn out. I was pleasantly surprised with the subtle complex flavors. Serve with shirataki noodles or rice, or cauliflower mash or just as it is.

MAKES 6 (4½-ounce) servings

2 tablespoons (30mL) coconut oil

4 chicken thighs and 4 chicken drumsticks, bone-in, skin-on, about 2¾ pounds (1.3Kg)

1 medium onion or shallot, diced

2 cloves garlic, minced

1 tablespoon (5.8g) almond flour

1 teaspoon (1.8g) ground coriander

¼ cup (60mL) chicken stock

1 (13½ oz, 400mL) can coconut milk with cream

2 teaspoons (12g) salt, plus more for seasoning

2 bay leaves

3 lime or orange leaves

2 lemongrass stalks, heavy ends bruised

1½-inch piece (9.8g) galangal or fresh ginger

freshly ground black pepper

PREPARE THE POT

1. Set the cooker to SAUTÉ, higher setting.

2. Once hot, melt the coconut oil.

3. Sprinkle a pinch each of salt and pepper on the chicken.

4. Brown the chicken in batches, about 2 to 3 minutes per side. Remove and set aside.

5. Add the onion and garlic, and sauté until the onion is soft, about 30 seconds.

6. Add the almond flour and coriander, and stir for 30 seconds to create a paste.

7. Pour in the stock and stir to deglaze the pot.

8. Stir in the coconut milk.

9. Add the salt, bay leaves, lime or orange leaves, lemongrass, and galangal or ginger.

10. Add the chicken, along with any drippings.

11. Close the lid and lock. SEAL the pressure valve.

12. Set to HIGH PRESSURE and cook for 14 minutes.

13. Then QUICK RELEASE.

14. Remove the citrus leaves, lemongrass, and galangal or ginger.

15. Spoon sauce over the top and serve.

VARIATION: I would love to try this recipe with Cornish game hens or lamb.

Nutrition Facts	
(amount per serving)	
Energy (calories)	556
Fat	43.5g
Protein	34.5g
Total Carbohydrates	6.7g
Fiber	0.7g
Net Carbohydrates	6g

Macronutrient Breakdown	
Fat	70.3%
Protein	24.8%
Carbs	4.8%

Salahub's Suspiciously Green Chicken Curry

This recipe was inspired by a colleague who used his slow cooker to make this dish for our holiday potluck. I had to do some revising for the pressure cooker, and also to make it a little more keto-friendly. The original recipe used six whole onions! It's a very mild but flavorful curry. The greenish tinge comes from the 2 tablespoons of coriander used. To soak up this sauce, serve with cauliflower rice, mashed cauliflower, shirataki noodles, or shirataki rice to help you get every last bit.

MAKES 12 servings, each 1 drumstick with sauce

Spices

1 teaspoon (3g) ground cumin

1 teaspoon (2.2g) ground cardamom

1 teaspoon (3g) ground turmeric

½ teaspoon (1g) ground cloves

1½ teaspoons (9g) salt

1 teaspoon (2.8g) cayenne pepper (if you like it hotter add ½ teaspoon more)

2 tablespoons (14.3g) ground coriander

Chicken

2 tablespoons (30mL) avocado oil or olive oil

2 cups (220g) onions, diced (about 2 medium onions)

2 cloves garlic, minced

1 tablespoon (12g) grated fresh ginger, or ½ tablespoon dried

1 cup (250mL) chicken stock or vegetable broth

1½ cups (375 mL) canned diced tomatoes with liquid

12 chicken drumsticks or thighs, bone-in, skin-on, about 3½ pounds (1.5kg)

1. Mix all of the spices together and set aside.

PREPARE THE POT

2. Set the pressure cooker to SAUTÉ.

3. Once hot, add the avocado oil or olive oil.

4. Add the onions and sauté until transparent, about 5 minutes.

5. Stir in the spice mix and stir for 1 to 2 minutes to toast and aromatize the spices.

6. Add the garlic and ginger, and sauté for 1 minute.

7. Pour in the stock and stir to deglaze the pot.

8. Add the tomatoes with their liquid.

9. Add the chicken.

10. Close the lid and lock. SEAL the pressure valve.

11. Set to HIGH PRESSURE and cook for 12 minutes.

12. Then QUICK RELEASE. Place a piece of chicken next to your favorite side and ladle the wonderful aromatic sauce over it. Enjoy!

VARIATIONS: Add 2 to 4 tablespoons of butter, cream, or coconut milk to add a little more depth and to bump up the fats. As mild as this curry is, using lamb or even mutton would work well.

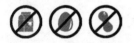

Nutrition Facts	
(amount per serving)	
Energy (calories)	251
Fat	15g
Protein	24.6g
Total Carbohydrates	3.6g
Fiber	1.2g
Net Carbohydrates	2.4g

Macronutrient Breakdown	
Fat	54%
Protein	40%
Carbs	6%

Satay Chicken

Chicken satay is normally grilled on skewers and then dipped in a small amount of sauce. In this recipe, the chicken really just serves as an excuse to eat more delicious peanut sauce.

MAKES 7 (¾-cup) servings

Sauce

1 (13½ oz, 400mL) can coconut milk with cream

2 tablespoons (30mL) apple cider vinegar

4 tablespoons (60g) natural peanut butter

2 tablespoons (30mL) fish sauce

1 tablespoon (15mL) liquid aminos

1 teaspoon (5mL) lime juice

Chicken

2 tablespoons (30mL) avocado oil

4 chicken thighs and 4 chicken drumsticks, bone-in, skin-on, about 2¾ pounds (1.3kg)

½ medium onion, chopped

1 teaspoon (6g) salt

1 whole star anise

1 red or green Thai chile pepper, split (add a second one for more heat)

½ cup (125mL) chicken stock

crushed peanuts, to serve

chopped cilantro, to serve

lime wedges, to serve

1. Whisk all the sauce ingredients together, removing any lumps. Set aside.

PREPARE THE POT

2. Set the pressure cooker to SAUTÉ.

3. When hot, add the avocado oil.

4. Brown the chicken in batches, then remove and set aside.

5. Add the onion and sprinkle with salt, and sauté until soft and translucent, about 1 ½ minutes.

6. Add the star anise and chile pepper. Sauté until fragrant, about 1 to 2 minutes.

7. Pour in the stock and stir to deglaze the pot.

8. Add the chicken pieces back to the pot, along with any drippings.

9. Pour the sauce over the top.

10. Set to HIGH PRESSURE and cook for 12 minutes.

11. Then MANUAL RELEASE PRESSURE after 2 to 3 minutes.

12. Remove the chicken pieces from the pot. Separate the meat from the bones and return the meat to the pot. Discard the bones or save for another use.

13. Serve with the sauce and garnish with peanuts, cilantro, and lime, if desired.

VARIATION: Try using chicken breast strips or beef strips. Not only would it bring about a different feel to the dish, but it would cut the cook time down to 6 to 10 minutes, depending on the size of the strip.

Nutrition Facts	
(amount per serving)	
Energy (calories)	443
Fat	37.3g
Protein	23.5g
Total Carbohydrates	5.6g
Fiber	0.7g
Net Carbohydrates	4.9g

Macronutrient Breakdown	
Fat	75%
Protein	21%
Carbs	5%

Double-Run Turkey Stock

During the holidays, I always make stock from the turkey carcass, but some years I have a pretty large carcass to work with. I noticed that after making stock once, or what I call the first run, there was still a lot of life left in the carcass, so I ran it a second time with fresh herbs. The first run was really amazing. The second run was still good! I used the second run of stock for the bases of dishes, whereas I used the first run of stock for drinking and soups. Essentially, just toss everything in the pot and let it go. And if you've still got company after the holidays, send them home with stock! Store stock in 1-quart (1L) Ziploc bags with the air removed, and pop in the freezer until you need it. If you have a pressure canner (this is different from a pressure cooker), you could can the stock too.

MAKES 3 to 3½ liters per run

1 turkey carcass from a 16-pound (7.4kg) turkey

1 turkey neck, uncooked

2 carrots, with skin, cut in thirds

3 stalks celery, with leaves, cut in thirds

1 medium onion, halved, with skin

½ head garlic, with skin

2 tablespoons (36g) salt, divided

6 to 8 sprigs fresh thyme, divided

4 sprigs fresh rosemary, divided

4 sprigs fresh sage, divided

PREPARE THE POT

1. Add everything to the pressure cooker, using only half the salt, thyme, rosemary, and sage.

2. Fill with cool water to 1 inch from the max-fill line.

3. Cover with the lid and lock. SEAL the pressure valve.

4. Set to HIGH PRESSURE and cook for 75 minutes.

5. Then let the pot NATURAL RELEASE pressure, about 15 minutes.

6. Pull out the inner pot, place on a hot pad, and carefully ladle stock through a strainer, leaving the solids in the pot.

7. If a second run is desired, continue on.

8. Add the remaining herbs and salt to the pot.

9. Place the inner pot back into the pressure cooker and fill back up with cool water to 1 inch from the max-fill line.

10. Set to HIGH PRESSURE and cook for 75 minutes.

11. Then let the pot NATURAL RELEASE pressure, about 15 minutes.

12. Strain the second run of stock to remove the solids.

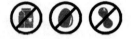

Nutrition facts and macronutrient breakdowns are not included for stocks and broths (see page 26).

Stewed Turkey

I'm used to only having turkey for holiday feasts, but I was surprised to see how often turkey parts are on sale. I wondered if it's possible to do Thanksgiving in a pot any time, especially when it's as simple as this! For a complete meal, serve with a side of green beans, Brussels sprouts, and low-carb cranberry sauce!

MAKES 4 (4½-ounce) servings

1 turkey drumstick and thigh, about 1¾ pounds, (791g), separated

¾ cup (180mL) chicken stock

½ medium onion, sliced

1 clove garlic, coarsely chopped

2 teaspoons (12g) salt

1 tablespoon (2g) dried sage

1 teaspoon (1.2g) dried rosemary

1 teaspoon (1g) dried thyme

1 bay leaf

¼ cup (½ stick, 56g) salted butter

freshly ground black pepper

PREPARE THE POT

1. Add all the ingredients to the pot.

2. Close the lid and lock. SEAL the pressure valve.

3. Set to HIGH PRESSURE and cook for 25 to 30 minutes.

4. Then QUICK RELEASE.

5. Remove the turkey and discard the bay leaf.

6. Shred the meat with two forks or cut into cubes, and pour the sauce over the top.

VARIATION: Not only could this be great with duck and squab, but also lamb, goat, and pork too.

Nutrition Facts	
(amount per serving)	
Energy (calories)	345
Fat	19.4g
Protein	39.9g
Total Carbohydrates	2.3g
Fiber	0.5g
Net Carbohydrates	1.8g

Macronutrient Breakdown	
Fat	50.6%
Protein	46%
Carbs	2.6%

Turkey Wing Vindaloo

I'd always wanted to make a vindaloo. I love the bold flavors, but I wasn't sure what to use until I stumbled upon a great special at my local butcher shop for turkey wings. You can absolutely use chicken in this recipe too, but it will rock with more strongly flavored meats. If you're not a fan of heat, I'd cut back on the cayenne and omit the chile pepper. If you can't find dried tamarind powder, just use ½ inch fresh, thinly sliced tamarind instead. Serve over cauliflower or cauliflower rice or broccoli mash, or even just steamed cauliflower or broccoli so the florets trap the delicious sauce.

MAKES 4 (4-ounce) servings

Spices

2 teaspoons (4.6g) paprika

2 teaspoons (4.2g) ground cumin

2 teaspoons (4g) ground mustard

2 teaspoons (3.6g) ground coriander

2 teaspoons (6g) ground turmeric

½ teaspoon (1.3g) ground cinnamon

1 teaspoon (2g) dried tamarind powder

1 teaspoon (1.8g) cayenne (for more heat, add ½ to 1 teaspoon more)

Turkey

2 tablespoons (25g) ghee

1¾ pounds (795g) turkey wings, about 4 wings, split and tips removed

1 large onion, diced

2 cloves garlic, minced

1 teaspoon (4g) grated fresh ginger

1 Thai chile, split (add a second chile for more heat)

1 bay leaf

½ cup (125mL) turkey or chicken stock

1 (28oz, 796mL) can diced tomatoes with liquid

1 tablespoon (15mL) white vinegar

sour cream or yogurt, to serve

1. Mix together the spices and set aside.

PREPARE THE POT

2. Set the pressure cooker to SAUTÉ.

3. Once hot, melt the ghee.

4. Brown the wings in batches, about 2 minutes each side, then set aside.

5. Add the onion, garlic, and ginger, and sauté until the onion is soft, about a minute.

6. Add the spice mix, chile, and bay leaf. Stir for about a minute to toast the spices.

7. Pour in the stock and stir to deglaze the pot.

8. Stir in the tomatoes and vinegar.

9. Add the wings, along with any of their juices.

10. Close the lid and lock. SEAL the pressure valve.

11. Set to HIGH PRESSURE and cook for 20 to 25 minutes.

12. Then QUICK RELEASE.

13. Remove the chile and bay leaf and discard.

14. Remove the wings and shred the meat with two forks. Set aside. Discard the bones or keep them for a future stock.

15. Blend the sauce in the pot with an immersion blender.

16. Return the turkey to the sauce.

17. Ladle into bowls.

VARIATIONS: If you need to cut the heat down a little, mix in some sour cream or yogurt. Vindaloo has a strong flavor and meats with a strong flavor benefit from this. Turkey thighs, pork, lamb, or goat are great alternatives.

DAIRY-FREE VARIATION: Make it dairy free by using coconut oil instead of ghee.

Nutrition Facts	
(amount per serving)	
Energy (calories)	383
Fat	23.1g
Protein	28.4g
Total Carbohydrates	15.3g
Fiber	6.5g
Net Carbohydrates	8.8g

Macronutrient Breakdown	
Fat	54%
Protein	30%
Carbs	16%

CHAPTER 6
Eggs

Spicy Egg Salad for One

One thing you learn quickly with the pressure cooker is that you can make an abundance of hard-boiled eggs that are super easy to peel. Hard-boiled eggs are good keto-friendly snacks to have on hand. I often cook half a dozen at a time and keep them in the fridge to eat as is or to make a quick egg salad. Scale up as needed.

MAKES 1 serving

2 eggs

2 tablespoons (27g) mayonnaise

½ teaspoon (2.5g) sriracha (add another ½ teaspoon for more heat)

1 teaspoon (2g) finely chopped green onions or chives

1 tablespoon (7.5g) finely chopped celery

salt

freshly ground pepper

PREPARE THE POT

1. Add 2 cups of water to the pot. Place the flat wire steam rack in the pot with the handle up.

2. Place the eggs directly on rack.

3. Close the lid and lock. SEAL the pressure valve.

4. Set to HIGH PRESSURE and cook for 5 minutes.

5. Then MANUAL RELEASE PRESSURE after 5 minutes.

6. Prepare an ice water bath in a bowl.

7. Remove the eggs, then place them in the ice water bath for 5 minutes.

8. Peel the eggs.

9. Mash the eggs with a fork and mix in the mayonnaise, sriracha, green onions or chives, and celery.

10. Add salt and pepper to taste.

VARIATION: Add ½ teaspoon curry powder, ¼ teaspoon dried, ground, chipotle pepper, and ¼ teaspoon ground mustard instead of the sriracha.

Nutrition Facts	
(amount per serving)	
Energy (calories)	325
Fat	30.7g
Protein	10.9g
Total Carbohydrates	1g
Fiber	0.2g
Net Carbohydrates	0.8g

Macronutrient Breakdown	
Fat	85%
Protein	13%
Carbs	1%

Poached Eggs

My husband loves poached eggs. One Sunday morning while making brunch, I wondered how well poached eggs would work in the pressure cooker, especially when you want to do a few at a time. He commented that the whites are fluffier when done in the pressure cooker than if they were poached on the stove.

MAKES 2 (2-egg) servings

butter, for greasing	salt
¾ cup water, divided	freshly ground pepper
4 eggs	

PREPARE THE POT

1. Add 1 cup of water to the pot. Place the flat wire steamer rack in the pot with the handle up.

2. Grease 4 half-cup ramekins generously with butter.

3. Add 3 tablespoons of water to each ramekin.

4. Crack 1 egg into each ramekin.

5. Sprinkle with a little salt and pepper.

6. Carefully place the ramekins, evenly spaced, on the steamer rack.

7. Cover with the lid and lock. SEAL the pressure valve.

8. Set to HIGH PRESSURE and cook for 4 minutes.

9. Then QUICK RELEASE.

10. Using mini silicone mitts, remove the ramekins from the pot.

11. Tip each ramekin to pour off the water.

12. Run a knife along the edge and tip out the egg.

VARIATION: Make egg cups using silicon cupcake holders. Line the cupcake holder with a thin slice of ham and crack an egg inside. Sprinkle cheese on top, along with some all-purpose seasonings that are sugar free such as Mrs. Dash or FlavorGod Everything Seasoning. Place cupcake holders onto steamer rack and cook as per directions above.

Nutrition Facts	
(amount per serving)	
Energy (calories)	143
Fat	9.51g
Protein	12.56g
Total Carbohydrates	0.7g
Fiber	0g
Net Carbohydrates	0.7g

Macronutrient Breakdown	
Fat	59%
Protein	35%
Carbs	2%

Cheesy Eggs

I gravitate to this dish when I'm craving an eggy, cheesy snack. I've always got eggs, cream, and Parmesan cheese on hand. It takes seconds to whip up; while it's cooking away I'll be cutting up an avocado to serve on top, along with a little salt.

MAKES 2 (½-cup) servings

butter, for greasing	¼ teaspoon (1.5g) salt
4 eggs	¼ cup (25g) grated Parmesan cheese
1 tablespoon (15mL) heavy cream, 33%	freshly ground pepper

PREPARE THE POT

1. Add 1 cup of water to the pot. Place the flat wire steamer rack in the pot with the handle up.

2. Grease a heatproof bowl that fits in the pressure cooker with butter.

3. Whisk together the eggs, cream, salt, Parmesan cheese, and a little pepper.

4. Pour the egg mixture into the prepared bowl. Cover the bowl with foil.

5. Cover with the lid and lock. SEAL the pressure valve.

6. Set to HIGH PRESSURE and cook for 4 minutes.

7. Then MANUAL RELEASE PRESSURE after 5 minutes.

8. Use mini silicone mitts to lift up the rack and carefully remove the bowl.

9. Cut the eggs into 2 servings before removing from the bowl.

VARIATIONS: Change up the cheese, such as with shredded aged cheddar and Swiss. Use different seasonings—there are some great mixed blends out there. Even a seasoning salt adds a little more flavor.

Nutrition Facts	
(amount per serving)	
Energy (calories)	197
Fat	14.2g
Protein	15.4g
Total Carbohydrates	1.2g
Fiber	0g
Net Carbohydrates	1.2g

Macronutrient Breakdown	
Fat	65%
Protein	31%
Carbs	2%

Ham and Eggs

This is perfect for brunch. Just whip everything together in a bowl and pop it in the pressure cooker! Just make sure to cut the ham pieces small. I usually serve this with sriracha for a little bit of heat.

MAKES 4 (½-cup) servings

butter, for greasing

6 eggs

¼ cup (60mL) heavy cream, 33%

1½ tablespoons (20g) butter, melted

¼ teaspoon (1.5g) salt

freshly ground pepper

¼ cup (25g) grated Parmesan cheese

1 tablespoon (15g) chopped onion

¼ cup (37.5g) small-diced ham

1 tablespoon (15g) shredded cheddar cheese (optional)

PREPARE THE POT

1. Add 1 cup of water to the pot. Place the flat wire steamer rack in the pot with the handle up.

2. Grease a heatproof bowl that fits in the pressure cooker with butter.

3. Whisk the eggs, then mix in the cream, melted butter, salt, pepper, Parmesan cheese, onion, and ham.

4. Pour the egg mixture into the prepared bowl. If desired, sprinkle a little bit of shredded cheddar cheese on top.

5. Cover the bowl with foil.

6. Cover with the lid and lock. SEAL the pressure valve.

7. Set to HIGH PRESSURE and cook for 20 minutes.

8. Then MANUAL RELEASE PRESSURE after 5 minutes.

9. Use mini silicone mitts to lift up the rack and carefully remove the bowl.

10. Cut the eggs into 4 servings before removing from the bowl.

VARIATION: This works well with sausage too. Just pick a sausage that is a little lean and make sure it's cooked beforehand. Then crumble it into the egg mixture before cooking.

Nutrition Facts	
(amount per serving)	
Energy (calories)	234
Fat	18.4g
Protein	12.8g
Total Carbohydrates	4.5g
Fiber	1.2g
Net Carbohydrates	3.3g

Macronutrient Breakdown	
Fat	70%
Protein	21%
Carbs	7%

CHAPTER 7

Pork and Lamb

Ham Bone Stock

I don't normally make a basic pork stock, but when I get my hands on a ham bone, you bet that's what I'm doing! I don't drink it as I do chicken broth, but instead just use it for stews. The yield for this stock will vary depending on the size of the ham bone.

MAKES about 2 liters

1 ham bone	3 stalks celery, cut in thirds
1 tablespoon (18g) salt	1 bay leaf
1 medium onion, skin on, halved	1 teaspoon (5mL) liquid smoke
2 carrots, cut in thirds	

PREPARE THE POT

1. Add all of the ingredients to the pot. Add enough water to just cover the ham bone by 1 inch.

2. Cover with the lid and lock. SEAL the pressure valve.

3. Set to HIGH PRESSURE and cook for 75 minutes.

4. Then MANUAL RELEASE PRESSURE after 10 minutes.

5. Store in the fridge for a week or transfer to Ziploc bags, remove the air, and store flat in the freezer for up to 3 months.

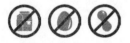

Nutrition facts and macronutrient breakdowns are not included for stocks and broths (see page 26).

Smoked Picnic Ham

For the holidays it's a feast at my family's place, and we usually have both ham and turkey. Since I got an Instant Pot, we don't have to worry about room in the oven for both the turkey and the ham. We now actually prefer cooking the ham in the pressure cooker to the oven.

MAKES 20 (2-ounce) servings

2 cups (500mL) pork or chicken stock

2 teaspoons (2.4g) dried rosemary

2 teaspoons (2g) dried thyme

5 pounds (2.3kg) fresh picnic ham, bone-in, smoked

Prepare the Pot

1. Add the stock, rosemary, and thyme to the pot.

2. Place in the flat wire steamer rack.

3. Set the ham on top of the rack.

4. Cover with the lid and lock. SEAL the pressure valve.

5. Set to HIGH PRESSURE and cook for 30 minutes.

6. Then QUICK RELEASE.

7. Check the internal temperature of the ham with an instant-read kitchen thermometer. It should read 145°F when done. If not, cook for an additional 5 to 10 minutes under HIGH PRESSURE until the internal temperature reads 145°F.

8. Once cooked, let rest for at least 3 to 5 minutes before carving.

9. Serve with the juices.

VARIATIONS: Instead of rosemary and thyme, use star anise and cloves. Use about 1 tablespoon of whole cloves and stud the ham.

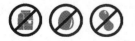

Nutrition Facts	
(amount per serving)	
Energy (calories)	335
Fat	35g
Protein	4g
Total Carbohydrates	0g
Fiber	0g
Net Carbohydrates	0g

Macronutrient Breakdown	
Fat	94%
Protein	5%
Carbs	0%

Farmer's Sausage and Cabbage Soup

When I was working on this recipe, I didn't realize that "farmer's sausage" can be a regional product. If you can't find it, just look for a smoked, cured pork sausage, and I'm sure it will work just fine. What I had in mind for this recipe was a borscht, but every family has their own distinct recipe that had been passed down for generations. So rather than step on toes, I opted not to call it by the name.

MAKES 12 (1-cup) servings

2 tablespoons (25g) bacon fat, ghee, or butter

1 medium onion, chopped

1 cup (86g) finely diced celery

1 cup (134g) finely diced carrot

2¼ teaspoons (13.5g) salt, divided

1 pound (454g) farmer's sausage, or other smoked, cured pork sausage, sliced into ½-inch coins

1 teaspoon (2.8g) coarsely ground pepper

2 teaspoons (3g) caraway seeds

⅓ cup (13g) fresh dill or 2 tablespoons (6.5g) dried dill, divided

1 medium cabbage, cored and diced large

4 cups (1L) pork, chicken, or vegetable stock

4 cups (1L) cool water

sour cream, to serve

PREPARE THE POT

1. Set the pressure cooker to SAUTÉ.

2. Once hot, the add bacon fat to melt.

3. Add in the onion, celery, and carrot. Sprinkle ¼ teaspoon of the salt over the top and sauté for 1 to 2 minutes until the onion is soft and translucent.

4. Add the sausage and cook for 2 minutes.

5. Add the remaining 2 teaspoons of salt along with the pepper, caraway, and half of the dill. Stir well.

6. Add the cabbage, stock, and water.

7. Cover with the lid and lock. SEAL the pressure valve.

8. Set to HIGH PRESSURE and cook for 12 minutes.

9. Then NATURAL RELEASE.

10. Season to taste with salt and pepper. Serve with a dollop of sour cream and the remaining dill.

VARIATION: Try using ground pork seasoned with hot and/or smoked paprika for a different spin on this dish.

Nutrition Facts	
(amount per serving)	
Energy (calories)	238
Fat	17.2g
Protein	10.7g
Total Carbohydrates	10.3g
Fiber	3.8g
Net Carbohydrates	6.5g

Macronutrient Breakdown	
Fat	64%
Protein	18%
Carbs	17%

Ham, Cabbage, and Black-Eyed Pea Soup

A wholesome, hearty soup for a chilly day.

MAKES 8 (1-cup) servings

2 tablespoons (30mL) avocado oil

1 medium onion, chopped

6 cups (1.5L) pork, chicken, or vegetable stock

1½ teaspoons (9g) salt

½ teaspoon (1.4g) coarsely ground black pepper

½ teaspoon (0.9g) ground cumin

½ teaspoon (0.9g) cayenne pepper

1 bay leaf

1 tablespoon (6.8g) paprika

1 tablespoon (9.6g) hickory spice blend (optional)

¼ cup (36g) dried black-eyed peas

1 (28oz, 796 mL) can diced tomatoes with liquid

½ head small cabbage, cored and shredded

1 teaspoon (1g) dried oregano

2 teaspoons (2g) dried thyme

1 to 1½ pounds (454g to 680g) ham, cubed, with fat

PREPARE THE POT

1. Set the pressure cooker to SAUTÉ.

2. Once hot, add the avocado oil.

3. Add the onion and sauté until translucent, about 1½ minutes.

4. Add the stock, salt, black pepper, cumin, cayenne, bay leaf, paprika, and hickory spice, if using.

5. Add the black-eyed peas.

6. Cover with the lid and lock. SEAL the pressure valve.

7. Set to HIGH PRESSURE and cook for 45 minutes.

8. Then QUICK RELEASE.

9. Add the tomatoes, cabbage, oregano, thyme, and ham.

10. Cover with the lid and lock. SEAL the pressure valve.

11. Set to HIGH PRESSURE and cook for 15 minutes.

12. Then QUICK RELEASE.

13. Ladle into bowls and serve.

VARIATION: For a faster soup, don't add the black-eyed peas. After sautéing the onions, just add in all the ingredients and cook on HIGH PRESSURE for 13 minutes then QUICK RELEASE.

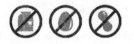

Nutrition Facts	
(amount per serving)	
Energy (calories)	194
Fat	11g
Protein	15.2g
Total Carbohydrates	8.8g
Fiber	3.1g
Net Carbohydrates	5.7g

Macronutrient Breakdown	
Fat	51%
Protein	31%
Carbs	18%

Hot Salami and Kale Soup

This recipe combines a few ingredients you might not think go together, but they do! This kitchen sink soup is deliciously keto.

MAKES 8 (1-cup) servings

2 tablespoons (25g) bacon fat

1 pound (454g) ground beef

¾ pound (340g) ground pork

2 cloves garlic, minced

1 medium onion, diced

1 cup diced fresh tomatoes

1 cup (28g) sliced celery

1 cup (47g) shredded kale

¾ cup (184g) sliced mushrooms

1 (28oz, 796 mL) can diced tomatoes, drained

4 cups (1L) chicken or beef stock

2 teaspoons (3.6g) dried oregano

6 slices hot Italian salami, sliced into strips

1 tablespoon (18g) salt

½ cup (72g) dried black-eyed peas

2 sprigs fresh thyme

1 bay leaf

⅔ cup (70g) grated Parmesan cheese

PREPARE THE POT

1. Set the pressure cooker to SAUTÉ.

2. When hot, add the bacon fat.

3. Add the ground beef and pork, break it apart, and brown for about 5 minutes.

4. Add the garlic and onion, and sauté for 1 minute. Then stir in the fresh tomatoes.

5. Add the celery, kale, and mushrooms. Let sit for 30 seconds then stir.

6. Add the canned tomatoes, stock, oregano, salami, salt, black-eyed peas, thyme, bay leaf, and Parmesan cheese, and stir to combine well.

7. Close the lid and lock. SEAL the pressure valve.

8. Set to HIGH PRESSURE and cook for 30 minutes.

9. Then NATURAL RELEASE.

10. Remove the thyme stems and bay leaf before serving.

VARIATIONS: Instead of kale, anything that's green and leafy works great, such as spinach, chile pepper leaves, and bok choy. Instead of ground beef and pork use ground turkey or chicken, and add poultry spices such as sage and rosemary in addition to the thyme.

Nutrition Facts	
(amount per serving)	
Energy (calories)	370
Fat	27.3g
Protein	18.1g
Total Carbohydrates	5.7g
Fiber	2.1g
Net Carbohydrates	3.61g

Macronutrient Breakdown	
Fat	72%
Protein	21%
Carbs	6%

Sausage, Kale, and Black-Eyed Pea Stoop

When it doesn't know if it's a stew or a soup, it's a stoop. This is wonderfully hearty and has a savory broth that doesn't disappoint. Great for those days when you're not sure if you want to zig or zag!

MAKES 7 (1-cup) servings

2 tablespoons (27g) ghee or butter

1 pound (454g) chorizo sausage, cut into ½-inch coins (about 5 sausages)

½ medium onion, chopped

2 cloves garlic, minced

1 teaspoon (2.1g) ground cumin

½ teaspoon (1.1g) hot paprika

2 teaspoons (12g) salt

½ teaspoon (1.4g) freshly ground pepper

2 cups (500mL) pork, chicken, or vegetable stock

1 can (28oz, 796 mL) diced tomatoes with liquid

½ cup (72g) dried black-eyed peas

½ cup (118mL) frozen peas and carrots

3½ cups (65g) chopped kale

1⅓ cups (180g) cubed zucchini

PREPARE THE POT

1. Set the pressure cooker to SAUTÉ.

2. Once hot, add the butter to melt.

3. Quickly brown the sausage, just 2 to 3 minutes, then remove from the pot.

4. Add the onion and garlic, and sauté until soft, about a minute.

5. Add the cumin, paprika, salt, and pepper. Stir for 30 seconds.

6. Pour about ½ cup of stock into the pot and stir to deglaze. Then add the rest of the stock.

7. Add the diced tomatoes with their liquid.

8. Add the black-eyed peas and the sausage along with its juices.

9. Close the lid and lock. SEAL the pressure valve.

10. Set to HIGH PRESSURE and cook for 60 minutes.

11. Then QUICK RELEASE.

12. Add the peas, carrots, kale, and zucchini.

13. Close the lid and lock. SEAL the pressure valve.

14. Set to HIGH PRESSURE and cook for 2 minutes.

15. Then MANUAL RELEASE PRESSURE after 1 minute.

16. Ladle into bowls.

VARIATIONS: If the black-eyed peas are a little too carby for your liking, omit them and add a little more zucchini or some cubed eggplant, along with some broccoli. Or if you're looking for more leafy goodness, chop up some baby bok choy and toss it in with the kale.

Nutrition Facts	
(amount per serving)	
Energy (calories)	273
Fat	19.9g
Protein	12.6g
Total Carbohydrates	11g
Fiber	4g
Net Carbohydrates	7g

Macronutrient Breakdown	
Fat	68%
Protein	19%
Carbs	16%

Zuppa Toscana

It's great chatting with people who love food as much as I do. Many of my friends will innocently ask if something is keto- or low carb–friendly because they are genuinely curious. When someone mentioned a soup from a popular restaurant chain, I thought, "I bet I could keto-ize that!" Substitute cauliflower in place of the orzo and get your friends to try it. I would normally make this with heavy cream but tried it with coconut milk for someone who's lactose intolerant, and was pleasantly surprised that it worked out so well! This recipe makes a lot, and is great for when you have company or for meal prep for the week.

MAKES 3½ liters, about 15 (1-cup) servings

2 slices bacon, cut into 1-inch pieces

1 pound (454g) Italian sausage, casings removed (about 5 sausages)

1 medium onion, chopped

2 cloves garlic, minced

2 cups (300g) diced ham

8 cups (2L) pork, vegetable, or chicken stock

1½ teaspoons (2.5g) red chile flakes, plus more to serve

1 teaspoon (1g) dried thyme

4 cups (354g) cauliflower florets

3 cups (50g) chopped kale, cut into strips

1 cup (250mL) coconut milk with cream or heavy cream, 33%

freshly grated Parmesan cheese, to serve

PREPARE THE POT

1. Set the pressure cooker to SAUTÉ.

2. Once hot, add the bacon and sausage meat. Stir for 2 to 3 minutes to brown the sausage.

3. Add the onion and garlic. Sauté with the meats for 30 seconds.

4. Stir in the ham, stock, red chile flakes, thyme, and cauliflower.

5. Close the lid and lock. SEAL the pressure release valve.

6. Set to HIGH PRESSURE and cook for 0 minutes just to bring it up to pressure, or set to LOW PRESSURE and cook for 5 minutes.

7. Then QUICK RELEASE.

8. Stir in the kale and coconut milk.

9. Set to WARM for 5 minutes before serving.

10. Season to taste. Serve with a sprinkle of red chile flakes and Parmesan cheese, if desired.

VARIATIONS: Use different greens such as mustard greens, pepper greens, or bok choy instead of kale. Omit the coconut milk or cream for a lighter soup.

DAIRY-FREE VARIATION: Use coconut milk and don't serve with Parmesan cheese.

Nutrition Facts	
(amount per serving)	
Energy (calories)	236
Fat	19.7g
Protein	10.1g
Total Carbohydrates	4.7g
Fiber	1.4g
Net Carbohydrates	3.3g

Macronutrient Breakdown	
Fat	76%
Protein	17%
Carbs	8%

Spaghetti Squash and Ham Tetrazzini

Spaghetti squash is a little higher in carbs than zucchini, which is what I usually use as a "pasta," but I wanted to change things up a little. Trying to fit in foods with a slightly higher carb count just takes a little meal planning for the day.

MAKES 6 (¾-cup) servings

1 medium spaghetti squash

2 tablespoons (27g) ghee, butter, or avocado oil, plus more for greasing

1 medium onion, diced

2 cloves garlic, minced

4 to 5 white mushrooms, sliced

1 cup (175g) cubed ham

¼ cup (60mL) chicken stock

1 teaspoon (6g) salt

⅔ cup (160mL) heavy cream 33%

1 cup (100g) grated Parmesan cheese, divided

red chile flakes, to serve

fresh ground pepper, to serve

fresh chopped parsley, to serve

1. Cut the spaghetti squash crosswise into 1½-inch rings. Scrape out the seeds.

PREPARE THE POT

2. Add 2 cups water and place in the flat wire steamer rack.

3. Place spaghetti squash rings on top of the rack.

4. Close the lid and lock. SEAL the pressure valve.

5. Set to HIGH PRESSURE and cook for 4 minutes.

6. Then QUICK RELEASE.

7. Remove squash with tongs.

8. Use a spoon or fork to remove the squash from the skin and set aside.

9. Clean the pot.

10. Set the pot to SAUTÉ.

11. Once hot, melt the ghee, butter, or avocado oil.

12. Add the onion and garlic and sauté until the onion becomes translucent, about 30 seconds.

13. Add the mushrooms and ham and stir to warm them up.

14. Pour in the stock and stir to deglaze the pot.

15. Add the salt, and whisk in the cream.

16. Stir in ½ cup of the Parmesan cheese.

17. Toss in the spaghetti squash and stir to combine.

18. Set the pressure cooker to WARM.

19. Let heat through for 1 to 3 minutes.

20. Meanwhile, grease 6 (2-cup) ovenproof dishes. Preheat the oven's broiler.

21. Divide the spaghetti squash mixture evenly among the dishes.

22. Sprinkle a tablespoon of the remaining ½ cup Parmesan cheese over each dish.

23. Place the dishes on a cookie sheet and pop them under the broiler.

24. Broil for 5 to 7 minutes or just until brown.

25. Garnish with red chile flakes, ground pepper, and parsley to serve, if desired.

VARIATIONS: Using canned tuna or salmon or a couple of poached chicken breasts (page 87) instead of ham makes this dish quick too.

Nutrition Facts	
(amount per serving)	
Energy (calories)	279
Fat	21.4g
Protein	12.5g
Total Carbohydrates	10.6g
Fiber	2.1g
Net Carbohydrates	8.5g

Macronutrient Breakdown	
Fat	68%
Protein	17%
Carbs	15%

Italian Sausages with Bell Peppers and Mushrooms

Not too long ago, I took a sausage-making class and found out that most sausages use pork shoulder meat, which has the perfect ratio of 15 percent of fat to meat, meaning it only takes a little bit of elbow grease and water to bind them. In chatting with a few participants, the makings of this recipe came to mind, and I did use the sausages I made in the class. Enjoy this on its own or on top of low-carb noodles.

MAKES 6 (1-cup) servings

2 tablespoons (25g) bacon fat, avocado oil, or olive oil

1 pound (454g) Italian sausages (4 or 5 sausages)

1 cup (160g) diced onion (about 1 medium)

2 cloves garlic, minced

1 red bell pepper, diced

1 yellow bell pepper, diced

8 white mushrooms, sliced

1 cup (250mL) pork, chicken, or vegetable stock

1 (28oz, 796 mL) can crushed tomatoes

¼ teaspoon (0.5g) red chile flakes (add ½ teaspoon for more heat)

1 tablespoon (2.1g) dried basil

1 teaspoon (1g) dried thyme

1 teaspoon (1g) dried oregano

1 bay leaf

2 teaspoons (12g) salt, plus more for seasoning

½ teaspoon (1.4g) freshly ground pepper

PREPARE THE POT

1. Set the pressure cooker to SAUTÉ.

2. When hot, add the bacon fat, avocado oil, or olive oil.

3. Brown the sausages, about 1 to 2 minutes per side. Remove and set aside.

4. Add the onion, garlic, peppers, and mushrooms. Sprinkle with a little salt and sauté for 1 minute.

5. Pour in the stock and stir to deglaze the pot.

6. Stir in the crushed tomatoes. Add the red chile flakes, basil, thyme, oregano, bay leaf, salt, and pepper. Stir to combine well.

7. Add the sausages back in along with any drippings.

8. Close the lid and lock. SEAL the pressure valve.

9. Set to HIGH PRESSURE and cook for 7 minutes.

10. Then QUICK RELEASE.

11. Remove the bay leaf before serving.

VARIATIONS: Instead of using Italian sausages, use chorizo, spicy if you like it. And instead of the basil, thyme, and oregano, use cumin, paprika, and cayenne.

Nutrition Facts	
(amount per serving)	
Energy (calories)	341
Fat	28.4g
Protein	12.8g
Total Carbohydrates	9.4g
Fiber	2.3g
Net Carbohydrates	7.1g

Macronutrient Breakdown	
Fat	75%
Protein	15%
Carbs	11%

Deconstructed Spring Rolls

The challenge for this particular dish is to cook it long enough to get the pressure cooker up high enough for the flavors to intermingle, but not so long that the greens become mushy. Low pressure setting to the rescue! Enjoy this straight from the bowl with a dash of liquid aminos or grab a lettuce leaf and wrap it up.

MAKES 6 (1-cup) servings

1 tablespoon (15mL) coconut oil or avocado oil

1 pound (454g) ground pork

1 medium onion, chopped

2 cloves garlic, minced

1 teaspoon (2g) grated fresh ginger

½ cup (125mL) chicken stock

¼ cup (60mL) liquid aminos

½ teaspoon (2.5mL) sesame oil

1 teaspoon (5mL) Worcestershire sauce

⅛ teaspoon (0.3g) Chinese five spice

1 teaspoon (5g) Swerve sweetener or erythritol

2 teaspoons (12g) sea salt

8 white mushrooms, sliced

1 cup (89g) shredded green cabbage

1 cup (76g) shredded red cabbage

1 heaping cup (102g) shredded bok choy

1 cup (83g) thinly sliced celery

sesame seeds, to serve

PREPARE THE POT

1. Set the pressure cooker to SAUTÉ.

2. Once hot, add the coconut oil or avocado oil.

3. Add the pork, break up, and brown, about 5 minutes.

4. When about half of the pork is browned, stir in the onion, garlic, and ginger.

5. Once all the pork is cooked, pour in the stock and stir to deglaze the pot.

6. Then stir in the liquid aminos, sesame oil, Worcestershire sauce, Chinese five spice, sweetener, salt, and mushrooms.

7. Close the lid and lock. SEAL the pressure valve.

8. Set to HIGH PRESSURE and cook for 2 minutes.

9. Then QUICK RELEASE.

10. Stir in the green and red cabbage, bok choy, and celery.

11. Close the lid and lock. SEAL the pressure valve.

12. Set to LOW PRESSURE and cook for 1 minute.

13. Then MANUAL RELEASE PRESSURE after 5 minutes.

14. Garnish with sesame seeds to serve.

VARIATIONS: For some variety, try adding a little jicama for texture and daikon to add some flavor. Use a variety of ground meats, such as beef, turkey, chicken, or lamb, for flavor variation.

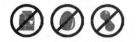

Nutrition Facts	
(amount per serving)	
Energy (calories)	271
Fat	21.2g
Protein	14.7g
Total Carbohydrates	6.1g
Fiber	1.7g
Net Carbohydrates	4.4g

Macronutrient Breakdown	
Fat	70%
Protein	22%
Carbs	9%

Kalua Pork

I asked a friend who grew up in Hawaii if she had a recipe for kalua pork. She didn't, but she had a friend who did! Feel free to wrap up the shoulder in banana leaves if you have access to them. This pork is excellent served with steamed cauliflower. After taking the pork out of the pressure cooker, toss a cauliflower head's worth of florets into the cooking liquid. Set to HIGH PRESSURE and cook for 0 minutes, just to bring it to pressure, then QUICK RELEASE.

MAKES 12 (4-ounce) servings

1½ cups (375mL) pork, chicken, vegetable stock

4½ pounds (2kg) pork picnic shoulder

1 tablespoon (15mL) hickory liquid smoke

4 teaspoons (24g) Hawaiian pink sea salt

PREPARE THE POT

1. Add the stock to the pressure cooker and set to SAUTÉ to warm it up while preparing the pork.

2. With a fork, poke holes all over pork roast. Drizzle with liquid smoke and sprinkle all over with pink sea salt.

3. Place the roast in warmed stock in the pressure cooker.

4. Close the lid and lock. SEAL the pressure valve.

5. Set to HIGH PRESSURE and cook for 90 minutes.

6. Then QUICK RELEASE.

7. The pork is done when it shreds easily with a fork. If not done to desired tenderness, set to HIGH PRESSURE for another 10 to 15 minutes and check again.

8. To speed up the process, cut the shoulder into 3 to 5 pieces, place it back in the pot, and set for 10 to 15 minutes.

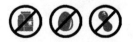

Nutrition Facts	
(amount per serving)	
Energy (calories)	322
Fat	20.8g
Protein	31.2g
Total Carbohydrates	0g
Fiber	0g
Net Carbohydrates	0g

Macronutrient Breakdown	
Fat	60%
Protein	40%
Carbs	0%

Korean-Inspired Pulled Pork

When I was putting this recipe together, I remembered a Korean classmate from high school saying, "Koreans like to sweat when they eat!" meaning they really like spicy food. I know this recipe will be nowhere near that level, but should you wish to add more chile paste, please do! Serve with some kimchi or on top of a bed of shredded cabbage to pick up the juices.

MAKES 12 (4-ounce) servings

Marinade

½ cup (125mL) liquid aminos

1 tablespoon (15g) Swerve sweetener or erythritol

2 teaspoons (10g) chili paste (also known as sambal oelek)

2 cloves garlic, smashed and peeled

1 teaspoon (5mL) Worcestershire sauce

⅛ teaspoon (0.5mL) sesame oil

1 teaspoon (5g) shrimp paste or 1 tablespoon (15mL) fish sauce

1 inch (2.5cm) fresh ginger, peeled and cut into matchsticks

Pulled Pork

3½ pounds (1.6kg) pork picnic shoulder

2 tablespoons (30mL) avocado oil

1 medium onion, chopped

1 teaspoon (6g) salt

1 cup (250mL) pork, chicken, or vegetable stock

1. Mix all the marinade ingredients in a large Ziploc bag, then add the pork shoulder. Seal and refrigerate for 1 to 2 hours, rotating the bag every half hour or so for the marinade to penetrate meat.

PREPARE THE POT

2. Set the pressure cooker to SAUTÉ. When hot, add the avocado oil and chopped onion. Sprinkle with salt.

3. Once the onion has become translucent and soft, about 1½ minutes, add the stock.

4. Remove the pork shoulder from the fridge and add to the pot, along with the marinade.

5. Close the lid and lock. SEAL the pressure valve.

6. Set to HIGH PRESSURE and cook for 90 minutes.

7. Then QUICK RELEASE.

8. The pork is done when it shreds easily with a fork. If not done to desired tenderness, set to HIGH PRESSURE for another 10 to 15 minutes and check again. To speed up the process, cut the shoulder into 3 to 5 pieces, place it back in the pot, and set for 10 to 15 minutes.

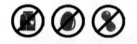

Nutrition Facts (amount per serving)	
Energy (calories)	300
Fat	20.1g
Protein	26.8g
Total Carbohydrates	1.2g
Fiber	0.2g
Net Carbohydrates	1g

Macronutrient Breakdown	
Fat	60.3%
Protein	35.7%
Carbs	1.6%

Spicy Pulled Pork

Pulled pork is always good. I used to cook it in my slow cooker with a bottle of barbecue sauce, but nowadays I do it in the pressure cooker. Now I'm looking to find other things to season the pork shoulder with that are vibrant enough to set off its succulent texture. Serve the pork in lettuce or a low-carb wrap, then top with a fried egg.

MAKES 12 (4-ounce) servings

Sauce

1 cup (250mL) sugar-free ketchup

juice of 1 lime

1 tablespoon (15g) Swerve sweetener or erythritol

1 tablespoon (8g) ancho chile powder

1 teaspoon (2.1g) ground cumin

1 teaspoon (1g) ground oregano

2 teaspoons (12g) salt

½ teaspoon (1.4g) freshly ground black pepper

Pulled Pork

2 tablespoons (30mL) avocado oil

3½ pounds (1.6kg) pork picnic shoulder

1 medium onion, chopped

1 teaspoon (6g) salt

2 cloves garlic, minced

1 cup (250mL) pork, chicken, or vegetable stock

1 can (4.2oz, 125mL) jalapeños, drained and chopped

1 can (7oz, 198g) chipotle peppers with adobo sauce

1 bunch cilantro, chopped, divided

fresh lime wedges for garnish

1. Mix all the sauce ingredients together and set aside.

PREPARE THE POT

2. Set the pressure cooker to SAUTÉ, higher setting.

3. Once hot, add the avocado oil.

4. Brown all sides of the pork shoulder, about 2 to 3 minutes on each side, then remove.

5. Add the onion, sprinkle with the salt, and sauté for 1 to 2 minutes, until soft.

6. Add the garlic, and stir for 30 seconds.

7. Pour in the stock and stir to deglaze the pot.

8. Stir in the mixed sauce ingredients from the first step, as well as jalapeños, chipotle peppers with their adobo sauce, and half the cilantro.

9. Add the pork back in along with any drippings. Spoon some of the liquid over the top.

10. Close the lid and lock. SEAL the pressure cooker.

11. Set to HIGH PRESSURE and cook for 90 minutes.

12. Then QUICK RELEASE. Vent the steam under a kitchen fan.

13. The pork is done when it shreds easily with a fork. If not done to desired tenderness, cook at HIGH PRESSURE for another 10 to 15 minutes and check again. To speed up the process, cut the shoulder into 3 to 5 pieces, place back in the pot, and cook for 10 to 15 minutes.

14. Serve with fresh lime juice and the remaining chopped cilantro.

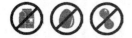

Nutrition Facts	
(amount per serving)	
Energy (calories)	354
Fat	23.9g
Protein	27g
Total Carbohydrates	6g
Fiber	1.3g
Net Carbohydrates	4.8g

Macronutrient Breakdown	
Fat	60%
Protein	30%
Carbs	7%

Pork Belly

I was inspired to create this dish when I came across a quick-cook pork belly at a popular retailer. For the price they were charging, and knowing that it usually takes at least a couple of hours to cook a pork belly in the oven, I knew I had to work on this one with the pressure cooker. Because pork belly is delicious and also high in fat, it falls nicely within the keto diet. Have a few sliced pieces with some hot sauce in a lettuce wrap like a taco.

MAKES 8 (2-ounce) servings

Rub

2 teaspoons (12g) sea salt

1 teaspoon (2.3g) paprika

¼ teaspoon (0.5g) cayenne pepper

¼ teaspoon (0.7g) freshly ground black pepper

Pork Belly

1 pound (454g) pork belly

1 tablespoon (15mL) liquid smoke (optional)

1. Mix the rub ingredients together and set aside.

2. Cut the pork belly into 1-inch-wide strips that fit in the pressure cooker.

3. Pat the rub all over the pork belly.

PREPARE THE POT

4. Add 1 cup of water to the pot along with the liquid smoke, if desired.

5. Put the flat wire steamer rack into the pot.

6. Place the pork belly pieces crosswise to the slots on the rack.

7. Close the lid and lock. SEAL the pressure valve.

8. Set to HIGH PRESSURE and cook for 60 minutes.

9. Then QUICK RELEASE.

10. Warm up a cast-iron pan over medium heat.

11. When it's nice and hot, place the pork belly pieces in fat-side down.

12. Let it crisp up for a few minutes, until nice and brown.

13. Then flip it over and crisp the other side.

14. Next, crisp the other two sides.

15. Remove from the pan and slice to serve.

VARIATION: Do the final cook step in the oven, under the broiler (it just may get a little smoky!) for 5 to 7 minutes or until crisp, or try it on the barbecue.

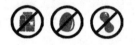

Nutrition Facts	
(amount per serving)	
Energy (calories)	295
Fat	30.1g
Protein	5.3g
Total Carbohydrates	0.2g
Fiber	0.1g
Net Carbohydrates	0.1g

Macronutrient Breakdown	
Fat	92%
Protein	5%
Carbs	0.3%

Pork Adobo

This was a Sunday afternoon dish in my household growing up. I could smell the peppercorns and bay leaves all afternoon. Little did I know at the time that pork adobo would be beneficial to my health. All I knew was that it's incredibly tasty! It was tough to get the recipe from my mother. All she said was, add the vinegar until it tastes "right." Gotta love recipes like that!

MAKES 14 (2-ounce) servings

1 medium onion, quartered

2 pounds (900g) pork belly, cut into 1-inch pieces

4 cloves garlic, unpeeled

¼ cup (60mL) liquid aminos

½ cup (125mL) apple cider vinegar

2 bay leaves

1 teaspoon (5mL) fish sauce (optional)

¼ inch (0.64cm) peeled, fresh ginger (optional)

2 tablespoons (30mL) avocado oil

1 cup (250mL) pork stock or water

1 teaspoon (2.3g) whole black peppercorns

1 teaspoon (6g) sea salt

1 teaspoon (4g) Swerve or erythritol

chopped green or spring onion, to serve

PREPARE THE POT

1. Add all of the ingredients to the pot.

2. Close the lid and lock. SEAL the pressure valve.

3. Set to HIGH PRESSURE and cook for 30 minutes.

4. Then MANUAL RELEASE PRESSURE after 10 minutes.

5. Remove the bay leaves, peppercorns, and ginger, if you added them.

6. Garnish with chopped green or spring onion.

VARIATION: Substitute chicken legs or another dark meat, and cook for 20 minutes.

TRADITIONAL VARIATION: Adobo is traditionally a mix of chicken and pork. So add the pork first, then after 10 minutes, release the pressure and add the chicken. Then cook for 20 minutes.

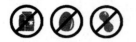

Nutrition Facts	
(amount per serving)	
Energy (calories)	360
Fat	36.4g
Protein	6.3g
Total Carbohydrates	1.5g
Fiber	0.2g
Net Carbohydrates	1.3g

Macronutrient Breakdown	
Fat	91%
Protein	7%
Carbs	1.6%

Pork Loin Steaks with Coconut Cream Sauce

Whenever I see boneless 7- to 10-pound pork loin roasts on sale, I'll pick a few up and cut one up into 1½- to 2-inch-thick steaks, the other into roasts and then freeze them all. They're a fast cook, as you can see by this 0-minute pressure cook time, as well as delicious and healthy.

MAKES 4 (6-ounce) servings, each 1 steak

2 tablespoons (27g) coconut oil

4 boneless 6-ounce (170g) pork loin steaks, 1½ to 2 inches thick

1 medium onion, sliced

⅔ cup (160mL) pork, chicken, or vegetable stock

2 teaspoons (12g) sea salt, plus more for seasoning

½ teaspoon (1.4g) freshly ground pepper, plus more for seasoning

3/4 cup (200mL) canned coconut milk with cream

1 tablespoon (1.8g) dried tarragon

1 tablespoon (5g) Dijon mustard (hot, if preferred)

PREPARE THE POT

1. Set the pressure cooker to SAUTÉ.

2. Once hot, add the coconut oil.

3. Season both sides of the pork loin steaks with salt and pepper.

4. Brown both sides of the steaks in two batches, 1 to 2 minutes on each side. Remove and set aside.

5. Add the onion and sauté until softened, about 1 minute.

6. Pour in the stock and stir to deglaze the pot.

7. Add the salt and pepper.

8. Whisk in the coconut milk, tarragon, and Dijon mustard. Add more coconut milk if desired.

9. Add the pork back into pot along with any drippings.

10. Close the lid and lock. SEAL the pressure cooker.

11. Set to HIGH PRESSURE and cook for 0 minutes just to bring it up to pressure.

12. Then QUICK RELEASE.

13. Remove the pork loin and set aside.

14. Set to SAUTÉ for 5 minutes while stirring occasionally to reduce sauce, if desired.

15. Drizzle the sauce over the pork to serve.

VARIATION: Instead of the tarragon and Dijon mustard, try 1 tablespoon of a mild curry powder.

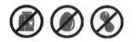

Nutrition Facts	
(amount per serving)	
Energy (calories)	502
Fat	38.4g
Protein	35g
Total Carbohydrates	4.2g
Fiber	0.6g
Net Carbohydrates	3.6g

Macronutrient Breakdown	
Fat	69%
Protein	28%
Carbs	3%

BBQ Pork Back Ribs

These ribs are a little thicker than side ribs and take just a little longer to cook, especially keeping them as half racks. Feel free to eat them right out of the cooker with the sauce, but I like to put them under the broiler or on the barbecue for less than 5 minutes a side to add a little bit of a charred flavor. Serve with coleslaw, if desired.

MAKES 6 (4-ounce) servings, about 2 ribs each

Sauce

1 cup (250mL) sugar-free ketchup

1 teaspoon (1.6g) onion flakes

2 teaspoons (10mL) cayenne pepper sauce (like Frank's Red Hot)

½ teaspoon (2.5mL) Worcestershire sauce

2 teaspoons (10mL) liquid aminos

¼ teaspoon (0.5g) garlic powder

½ teaspoon (0.5g) dried oregano

½ teaspoon (2.5g) Swerve sweetener or erythritol

½ teaspoon (2.5mL) apple cider vinegar

1 tablespoon (15mL) butter, melted

Pork Back Ribs

2¼ pounds (1 kg) pork back ribs (about 12 ribs)

1 to 2 teaspoons (12g) salt

½ teaspoon (1.4g) freshly ground pepper

1. Mix together all the sauce ingredients and set aside.

PREPARE THE POT

2. Add 2 cups of water to the pot and place in the flat wire steamer rack.

3. Cut the rib rack in half. Sprinkle both sides with salt and pepper.

4. Place the ribs upright on the steamer rack.

5. Close the lid and lock. SEAL the pressure valve.

6. Set to HIGH PRESSURE and cook for 20 minutes. If you want the meat to fall off the bone, cook for 25 minutes.

7. Then QUICK RELEASE.

8. Remove the ribs with tongs. Preheat the oven's broiler.

9. Remove a tablespoon of the steaming water from the pot and whisk it into the sauce.

10. Spread about ⅓ cup of sauce on the underside and sides of ribs.

11. Place the ribs on a foil-lined cookie sheet or on a broiler rack, underside up.

12. Broil for 4 minutes.

13. Take them out of the oven, flip, and spread ⅓ cup of sauce on the tops. If you don't want to use the extra sauce for dipping, slather the rest of it on.

14. Place the ribs back under the broiler for another 4 to 5 minutes.

15. Remove from the oven and serve with extra sauce.

Nutrition Facts	
(amount per serving)	
Energy (calories)	297
Fat	20.4g
Protein	22.5g
Total Carbohydrates	3g
Fiber	0.1g
Net Carbohydrates	2.9g

Macronutrient Breakdown	
Fat	62%
Protein	30%
Carbs	4%

Pork Side Ribs

This recipe is for those times when you've got a craving for ribs and want them pretty quick!

MAKES 6 (4-ounce) servings, about 2 ribs each

Sauce

1 cup (250mL) sugar-free ketchup

1 tablespoon (15g) Swerve sweetener

½ teaspoon (2.5mL) maple extract

2 teaspoons (10mL) liquid smoke

1 teaspoon (2.3g) paprika (use hot if you'd like)

1 teaspoon (6g) salt

¼ teaspoon (0.5g) ground pepper

Pork Side Ribs

2¼ pounds (1kg) pork side ribs (about 12 ribs)

2 tablespoons (27g) bacon fat or olive oil
½ cup (125mL) pork, chicken, or vegetable stock, or water

salt

freshly ground pepper

1. Whisk together all sauce ingredients and set aside.

2. Cut all the ribs apart.

3. Season with salt and pepper

PREPARE THE POT

4. Set the pressure cooker to SAUTÉ.

5. Once hot, add the bacon fat or olive oil.

6. Brown the ribs in batches and set aside.

7. Remove any excess oil from pot.

8. Pour in the stock and stir to deglaze the pot.

9. Add the ribs and half of the sauce.

10. Close the lid and lock. SEAL the pressure valve.

11. Set to HIGH PRESSURE and cook for 11 minutes. If you want the meat to fall off the bone, cook for 13 minutes.

12. Then NATURAL RELEASE.

13. Take the ribs out and toss with the rest of sauce.

VARIATION: For some heat, mix in some cayenne pepper sauce or some smoky heat, such as the adobo sauce from a can of chipotle chiles.

Nutrition Facts	
(amount per serving)	
Energy (calories)	380
Fat	30.9g
Protein	18.4g
Total Carbohydrates	2.9g
Fiber	0.1g
Net Carbohydrates	2.8g

Macronutrient Breakdown	
Fat	73%
Protein	19%
Carbs	3%

Lamb Stew

I wasn't really a fan of lamb, but thought I should give it another try. I used Australian lamb for this recipe, which may or may not have made a difference, but I was pretty pleased with how it turned out.

MAKES 5 (1-cup) servings

2 tablespoons (25g) ghee

1 pound (454g) lamb stew pieces, about 1-inch each

1 medium onion, chopped

2 cloves garlic, minced

½ cup (125mL) lamb or vegetable stock, or water (add ¼ to ½ cup more if you want it saucier)

2 tablespoons (16g) tomato paste

1 (28oz, 796mL) can diced tomatoes with liquid

½ teaspoon (0.5g) dried thyme

½ teaspoon (0.7g) dried summer savory

1½ teaspoons (1.8g) dried rosemary

1 bay leaf

2 teaspoons (12g) salt, plus more for seasoning

½ teaspoon (1.4g) freshly ground pepper, plus more for seasoning

1 medium stalk celery, diced

1 heaping cup (114g) cauliflower florets

10 white mushrooms, quartered

½ cup (70g) frozen peas and carrots

PREPARE THE POT

1. Set the pressure cooker to SAUTÉ.

2. Once hot, add the ghee.

3. Season the lamb with salt and pepper.

4. Brown the lamb pieces, then remove and set aside.

5. Add the onion, and sauté until soft, about 1 minute, then add the garlic.

6. After 30 seconds, pour in the stock and stir to deglaze the pot.

7. Whisk in the tomato paste, then add the diced tomatoes along with their liquid.

8. Stir in the thyme, savory, rosemary, bay leaf, salt, and pepper.

9. Add the lamb along with any drippings.

10. Close the lid and lock. SEAL the pressure cooker.

11. Set to HIGH PRESSURE and cook for 7 minutes.

12. Then QUICK RELEASE.

13. Stir in the celery, cauliflower, mushrooms, and peas and carrots.

14. Set to HIGH PRESSURE and cook for 0 minutes just to bring it up to pressure.

15. Then QUICK RELEASE.

16. Ladle into bowls.

DAIRY-FREE VARIATION: Replace ghee with avocado oil.

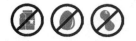

Nutrition Facts	
(amount per serving)	
Energy (calories)	312
Fat	20.6g
Protein	25g
Total Carbohydrates	7.2g
Fiber	2.1g
Net Carbohydrates	5.1g

Macronutrient Breakdown	
Fat	59%
Protein	32%
Carbs	9%

Shepherd's Pie

This was my first real shepherd's pie. I had always made them with beef, never lamb. Both my husband and I aren't normally fans of lamb, but this dish won us over.

MAKES 4 to 6 (1-cup) servings

2 tablespoons (25g) ghee or butter

1 medium onion, chopped

2 cloves garlic, minced

1 pound (454g) ground lamb

1 teaspoon (6g) salt

¾ teaspoon (2.1g) freshly ground pepper

5 white mushrooms, sliced

¼ cup (35g) frozen peas and carrots

½ cup (125mL) sugar-free ketchup

1 tablespoon (15mL) Worcestershire sauce

2 tablespoons (30mL) heavy cream, 33%

3 cups Cauliflower Mash (page 186)

1 cup (113g) shredded cheddar cheese

PREPARE THE POT

1. Set the pressure cooker to SAUTÉ.

2. Once hot, add the ghee or butter.

3. Add the onion and sauté for 1 to 2 minutes until soft. Add the garlic, and stir for 30 seconds.

4. Add the ground lamb, sprinkle the salt and pepper over the top, and brown.

5. Add the mushrooms and stir for about a minute.

6. Add the peas and carrots, ketchup, Worcestershire sauce, and cream. Stir to combine.

7. Close the lid and lock. SEAL the pressure valve.

8. Set to HIGH PRESSURE and cook for 1 minute.

9. Then QUICK RELEASE.

10. Transfer the meat into 4 to 6 heatproof individual dishes that fit into the pressure cooker. Cook in batches if needed. Divide the cauliflower mash evenly among the dishes over the top of the lamb filling.

11. Cover the dishes with foil.

12. Clean the pot.

13. Add 2 cups of water to the pot and place in the flat wire steamer rack.

14. Place the containers on the wire rack.

15. Set to HIGH PRESSURE and cook for 5 minutes.

16. Then QUICK RELEASE.

17. Carefully remove the dishes from the pot. Preheat the oven's broiler.

18. Remove the foil and top the shepherd's pies with cheddar cheese.

19. Place on a foil-lined cookie sheet and place under the broiler for 2 to 3 minutes, until the cheese is melted.

VARIATION: Lamb may not be everyone's cup of tea, so make it a cottage pie and substitute ground beef or a mix of beef with pork.

Nutrition Facts	
(amount per serving)	
Energy (calories)	491
Fat	39.1g
Protein	21.9g
Total Carbohydrates	13.7g
Fiber	4.1g
Net Carbohydrates	9.6g

Macronutrient Breakdown	
Fat	71%
Protein	17%
Carbs	11%

CHAPTER 8
Fish and Seafood

Moqueca (Brazilian Fish Stew)

Coconut oil contains medium-chain triglycerides (MCTs), which are good fats for the ketogenic diet. Palm oil does too, but it's not as easy to obtain compared to coconut oil. This dish is known in some parts of Brazil for its characteristic red-orange color imparted by the palm oil. Some cooks who have been unable to obtain palm oil added food color to their dish! If ocean friendly, sustainable basa fish isn't available in your area, find a nice firm white fish with subtle flavor such as cod, haddock, or tilapia.

MAKES 4 to 6 (¾-cup) servings

Marinade

2 cloves garlic, crushed

juice of 1 lime

½ teaspoon (3g) sea salt

¼ teaspoon (0.7g) freshly ground black pepper

Stew

1 pound (454g) basa filets, cut into 1-inch strips crosswise

2 tablespoons (27g) palm oil

1 medium onion, chopped

1½ cups (142g) diced red bell pepper (or a combination of red, orange, and yellow)

1½ cups (285g) diced tomatoes

1 cup (250mL) coconut milk with cream

2 teaspoons (2.3g) paprika

2 teaspoons (2.1g) ground cumin

1 teaspoon (1.8g) cayenne pepper

2 teaspoons (12g) salt

½ teaspoon (1.4g) freshly ground black pepper

chopped green onion or chives, to serve

lime wedges, to serve

1. Mix together the marinade ingredients, then add the fish. Cover and let marinate in the fridge for 20 minutes.

PREPARE THE POT

2. Set the pressure cooker to SAUTÉ.

3. Once hot, melt the palm oil.

4. Add the onion and red pepper, and sauté until soft, about 5 minutes.

5. Add the tomatoes and cook until broken down, about 2 to 3 minutes.

6. Stir in the coconut milk.

7. Stir in the paprika, cumin, cayenne pepper, salt, and black pepper.

8. Add in the fish along with the marinade.

9. Close the lid and lock. SEAL the pressure valve.

10. Set to HIGH PRESSURE and cook for 0 minutes, just to bring it up to pressure.

11. Then MANUAL RELEASE PRESSURE after 1 to 2 minutes.

12. Garnish with chopped green onions or chives, and lime wedges to serve.

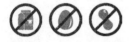

Nutrition Facts	
(amount per serving)	
Energy (calories)	368
Fat	27.4g
Protein	20.1g
Total Carbohydrates	10.3g
Fiber	2.5g
Net Carbohydrates	7.8g

Macronutrient Breakdown	
Fat	67%
Protein	22%
Carbs	11%

Cheesy Tuna Eggs

Whether it's breakfast, brunch, or even dinner, eggs are great all the time. It's simple to scramble some eggs, toss them in a bowl with some omelet fixings, and pop them into the pressure cooker while working on something else, like cooking bacon.

MAKES 4 (½-cup) servings

butter, for greasing

6 eggs, beaten

2 tablespoons (30mL) heavy cream, 33%

1 (5.8oz, 165g) can tuna packed in water, drained and flaked

1 teaspoon (1.6g) onion flakes

¼ teaspoon (1.5g) salt

⅛ teaspoon (0.5g) freshly ground pepper

¼ cup (25g) grated Parmesan cheese

PREPARE THE POT

1. Add 2 cups of water to the pot. Place in the flat wire steamer rack with the handle up.

2. Grease a heatproof bowl that fits in the pressure cooker with butter.

3. Whisk together the eggs, cream, tuna, onion flakes, salt, pepper, and Parmesan cheese.

4. Pour into the buttered bowl. Cover with foil and place on the rack.

5. Close the lid and lock. SEAL the pressure valve.

6. Set to HIGH PRESSURE and cook for 20 minutes.

7. Then MANUAL RELEASE PRESSURE after 5 minutes.

8. Use mini silicone mitts to lift up rack and carefully remove the bowl.

9. Cut into 4 servings before removing the eggs from the bowl.

VARIATIONS: Use canned salmon or ham instead of tuna. Try adding in some herbs such as dill, chives, or parsley.

Nutrition Facts	
(amount per serving)	
Energy (calories)	210
Fat	11.3g
Protein	25.8g
Total Carbohydrates	0.9g
Fiber	0g
Net Carbohydrates	0.9g

Macronutrient Breakdown	
Fat	48%
Protein	49%
Carbs	1.7%

Pesto Mussels

The toughest part of this dish is cleaning the mussels. It's great as a main dish for one or two or as an appetizer for a few. Enjoy as is with some chopped fresh tomatoes and basil, or serve on top of low-carb noodles.

MAKES 2 (1½-cup) servings

2 tablespoons (25g) ghee

½ medium onion, sliced

2 cloves garlic, coarsely chopped

½ cup (125mL) cool water

2 teaspoons (12g) sea salt

½ teaspoon (1.4g) freshly ground pepper

2 tablespoons (32g) prepared pesto

1 pound (454g) fresh mussels in shell, cleaned and beards removed and 25% yield (about 20 to 25 mussels)

chopped fresh basil, to serve

fresh chopped tomatoes, to serve

PREPARE THE POT

1. Set the pressure cooker to SAUTÉ.

2. Once hot, melt the ghee.

3. Add the onion and sauté until soft, about 1½ minutes.

4. Then add the garlic and sauté until aromatic, about 30 seconds.

5. Add the water, salt, pepper, and pesto, and stir to combine well.

6. Mix in the mussels.

7. Close the lid and lock. SEAL the pressure valve.

8. Set to HIGH PRESSURE and cook for 0 minutes, just to bring it up to pressure.

9. Then QUICK RELEASE.

10. Transfer the mussels into bowls.

11. Ladle sauce on top and garnish with chopped fresh basil and tomatoes, and a little freshly ground pepper.

VARIATION: Add in or substitute the mussels with clams, shrimp, or prawns.

DAIRY-FREE VARIATION: Replace ghee with avocado oil.

Nutrition Facts	
(amount per serving)	
Energy (calories)	331
Fat	29.8g
Protein	10.2g
Total Carbohydrates	7.8g
Fiber	1.4g
Net Carbohydrates	6.4g

Macronutrient Breakdown	
Fat	78%
Protein	12%
Carbs	9%

Poached Salmon Two Ways

Here's a set of recipes for people who are looking for ideas to meal prep. The cooking method is the same, but the recipes for the marinades are different. They're a little subtle in flavor so you can be sure to taste the fish. You can increase the number of filets; just make sure that there's enough room so that they're all touching the bottom of the pot. Watch out for thicker filets, over 1 inch (2.5cm) thick, as they may need a little longer to cook through before releasing the pressure. Greens such as bok choy, kale, spinach, broccoli, and green beans are nice accompaniments. Just add some good fats in there.

MAKES 1 (4-ounce) serving

Marinade 1: Asian-Inspired

3 tablespoons (45mL) liquid aminos

1-inch fresh ginger (2.5cm) cut into matchsticks

⅛ teaspoon (0.5mL) sesame oil

1 clove garlic, peeled and smashed

⅛ teaspoon (0.63g) red chile flakes

Marinade 2: Limey Dill

½ teaspoon (2.5g) lime zest

1 tablespoon (15g) fresh dill

½ (2.5g) teaspoon salt

Salmon

1 fresh salmon filet (4oz, 113g)

1. Mix the ingredients for your marinade of choice in a small Ziploc bag. Add the fish and refrigerate for 1 hour.

PREPARE THE POT

2. Add 1 cup of water to the pressure cooker.

3. Place the fish directly in the pot, making sure that it's touching the bottom.

4. Pour the marinade over the top of the fish.

5. Close the lid and lock. SEAL the pressure valve.

6. Set to HIGH PRESSURE cook for 0 minutes, just to bring it up to pressure.

7. Then MANUAL RELEASE PRESSURE after 1 minute.

8. Check to make sure the fish is done. The fish should look opaque and not glassy throughout. If not, repeat step 6.

9. Remove from the pot and let rest for about a 1 minute before serving.

VARIATION: Another alternative to marinating the salmon is flavoring the poaching liquid. Dill is always a great choice.

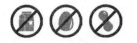

Nutrition Facts	
(amount per serving)	
Energy (calories)	144
Fat	5g
Protein	23g
Total Carbohydrates	0g
Fiber	0g
Net Carbohydrates	0g

Macronutrient Breakdown	
Fat	32%
Protein	67%
Carbs	0%

Salmon Alfredo Zoodles

Salmon is such a beautiful, tasty fish. It's a little oily, which provides those wonderful omega-3 fatty acids. I was missing salmon, capers, and cream cheese on a bagel recently and wondered if they would work together in a zoodles dish, and they do! You can omit the capers if they're not your thing. Serve with grated Parmesan cheese, fresh dill, and freshly ground pepper.

MAKES 6 (1-cup) servings

2 tablespoons (28g) ghee, butter, or avocado oil

½ medium onion, finely chopped

1 clove garlic, minced

1 pound (454g) salmon filet, about 2 inches thick, skin and bones removed

1 cup (250g) fish/seafood or vegetable stock, or water

¼ cup (62.5g) plus 1 tablespoon (15g) fresh dill, divided

2 teaspoons (12g) salt

¾ cup (180mL) heavy cream, 33%

2 tablespoons (29g) cream cheese, cubed

¾ cup (75g) grated Parmesan cheese

2 medium zucchini, spiralized or grated

2 tablespoons (17.2g) capers, drained and rinsed (optional)

salt

freshly ground pepper

PREPARE THE POT

1. Set the pressure cooker to SAUTÉ.

2. Once hot, melt the ghee, butter, or avocado oil.

3. Add the onion and garlic and sauté until the onion is soft, about 1 minute.

4. Place salmon on the bed of onions, let sit for 1 to 2 minutes, then flip over.

5. Add stock or water, 1 tablespoon of the dill, and the salt.

6. Close the lid and lock. SEAL the pressure valve.

7. Set to HIGH PRESSURE and cook for 0 minutes, just to bring it up to pressure.

8. Then RELEASE after 1 minute.

9. Carefully remove the salmon and set aside.

10. Set the pressure cooker to SAUTÉ.

11. Once the liquid is just bubbling, whisk in the cream.

12. Whisk in the cream cheese, then the Parmesan cheese.

13. Stir in the spiralized or grated zucchini.

14. Cover the pot and set to WARM.

15. Let heat through for 1 to 3 minutes or until the zoodles are at the desired consistency.

16. Cut or lightly shred the salmon into small, bite-sized pieces.

17. Then, in the pressure cooker, gently mix in the salmon along with any drippings, the remaining ¼ cup dill, and the capers, if using. Season with salt and pepper to taste.

VARIATION: To enjoy this as chowder, omit the zoodles and add a little more stock along with some cauliflower and other seafood such as clams or shrimp.

Nutrition Facts	
(amount per serving)	
Energy (calories)	394
Fat	31.1g
Protein	23.1g
Total Carbohydrates	6.3g
Fiber	1.4g
Net Carbohydrates	4.9g

Macronutrient Breakdown	
Fat	71%
Protein	23%
Carbs	6%

Seafood Stew

Calling all seafood fans: This is one recipe you'll definitely want to make! The hardest part is cleaning the mussels beforehand. For the fish filet, be sure to choose a firm white fish like cod, basa, haddock, or tilapia.

MAKES 7 to 8 (1-cup) servings

2 tablespoons (25g) ghee

½ medium onion, sliced

2 cups (380g) chopped fresh tomatoes

2 cloves garlic, minced

1 cup (255g) canned diced tomatoes with liquid

1 cup (250mL) coconut milk with cream

1 tablespoon (16g) tomato paste

1 cup (250mL) fish/seafood or vegetable stock, or cool water

1 to 2 bay leaves

2 teaspoons (12g) salt

½ teaspoon (1.4g) freshly ground pepper

1 pound (454g) fresh mussels in shell, cleaned and beards removed

1 pound (454g) fresh clams in shell, cleaned

2 cups (232g) prawns or shrimp, shell-on, fresh or frozen and thawed

2 cups (264g) cubed fish filet, in 2-inch cubes

chopped fresh cilantro, to serve

lemon wedges, to serve

Prepare the Pot

1. Set the pressure cooker to SAUTÉ.

2. Once hot, melt the ghee.

3. Add the onion and sauté until soft, about 1½ minutes.

4. Add the fresh tomatoes, stir, and let heat up for 2 minutes.

5. Stir in the garlic.

6. Add the canned tomatoes, coconut milk, tomato paste, and stock or water, and stir to combine.

7. Add the bay leaf, salt, and pepper, and stir to combine.

8. Add the mussels, clams, shrimp, and fish filet, and stir.

9. Cover with the lid and lock. SEAL the pressure valve.

10. Set to HIGH PRESSURE and cook for 0 minutes just to bring it up to pressure.

11. Then QUICK RELEASE.

12. Ladle into bowls and garnish with cilantro, lemon wedges, and a little freshly ground pepper.

VARIATIONS: Try using other types of shellfish such as crab legs, scallops, or shelled oysters. Add some green leafy vegetables such as baby bok choy, spinach, and kale along with the seafood. That short cooking process will have them just cooked and retaining a little crispness.

DAIRY-FREE VARIATION: Replace ghee with avocado oil.

Nutrition Facts	
(amount per serving)	
Energy (calories)	191
Fat	12.6g
Protein	13.4g
Total Carbohydrates	6.2g
Fiber	1.5g
Net Carbohydrates	4.7g

Macronutrient Breakdown	
Fat	59%
Protein	28%
Carbs	12%

Spicy Coconut Prawns

There's a good chance that you don't have shellfish stock lying around. Not to worry, I didn't either. I remember from my childhood my mom boiling shells from shrimp and using the water in other dishes. I think she added a few other things to make the stock, but it was really flavorful from the shells alone. Now I try to pick up shrimp with the shells on just so I can remove them to use them for stock. You can make this recipe without the stock, but it does add a little more depth to the dish.

MAKES 3 to 4 (½-cup) servings

Prawn Stock

1½ cups (375mL) cool water

1 pound (454g) prawns/shrimp, deveined

Coconut Prawns

2 tablespoons (30mL) coconut oil

½ cup (55g) chopped onion

2 cloves garlic, minced

1 small chile pepper, hot, chopped (add a second chile for more heat)

1 teaspoon (6g) sea salt

1 cup (250mL) coconut milk with cream

2 tablespoons (30mL) lemon juice, from about 1 lemon

½ teaspoon (0.5g) dried thyme

½ teaspoon (1.3g) ground cinnamon

chopped fresh cilantro, to serve

chopped fresh tomatoes, to serve

PREPARE THE POT

1. To make a super-simple, quick stock base, remove the shells from the shrimp or prawns and set the meat aside. Add the water and shells to the pot.

2. Set to SAUTÉ.

3. Let boil for 5 minutes or so, then turn the pressure cooker off.

4. Let cool. Remove the shells and transfer the stock to another container.

5. Set the pressure cooker to SAUTÉ. When hot, add the coconut oil.

6. Add the onion and sauté until softened, about 1 minute.

7. Next stir in the garlic and chile pepper. Sprinkle in the salt. Sauté for about 15 seconds or just until aromatic.

8. Add the prawn stock, coconut milk, and lemon juice.

9. Whisk in the thyme and cinnamon.

10. Add the prawn meat.

11. Close the lid and lock. SEAL the pressure valve.

12. Set to HIGH PRESSURE and cook for 0 minutes just to bring it up to pressure.

13. Then QUICK RELEASE.

14. Spoon into bowls and serve with chopped cilantro and tomatoes, if desired.

VARIATION: The flavors used in this dish would work well for a delicate-flavored white fish too, such as tilapia, basa, and probably even cod. Use filets and cut into cubes.

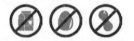

Nutrition Facts	
(amount per serving)	
Energy (calories)	265
Fat	20.2g
Protein	17g
Total Carbohydrates	5.8g
Fiber	0.7g
Net Carbohydrates	5.1g

Macronutrient Breakdown	
Fat	66%
Protein	25%
Carbs	8%

Steamed Basa Fish Filet Packets

In my travels I've seen athletes become ketogenic for a couple of weeks to a month before their sporting events. Seeing their meal preps inspired me for this recipe that's quick, easy, and simple to alter for a variety of flavors. As it's a clean and simple flavor profile, serving it with a side of green beans or Brussels sprouts or on top of a salad with a dill dressing would coordinate nicely. Or simply serve with fresh dill and lemon.

MAKES 2 (5.5oz) servings, 1 filet each

2 5-ounce filets (159g) basa fish

½ teaspoon (3g) salt

freshly ground pepper

1½ tablespoons (21g) butter, plus a little for greasing

1 tablespoon chopped fresh dill

2 or 3 lemon wedges

PREPARE THE POT

1. Add 1½ cups of water to the pressure cooker.

2. Place in the flat wire steamer rack.

3. Season the filets with salt and pepper on both sides.

4. Cut a sheet of foil to about twice the width of a piece of paper (about 17 inches).

5. Grease the center of the foil with additional butter.

6. Place filets on the center. It's okay if they overlap a little.

7. Place the butter in the middle and sprinkle the dill all over.

8. Lay the lemon slices spaced out evenly on top.

9. Seal up the foil, so that the seam is on top. Fold up the ends.

10. Place the packet seam-side up in the middle of the rack. Try to position it so that the ends don't touch the sides of the pan.

11. Set to HIGH PRESSURE and cook for 6 minutes.

12. Then MANUAL RELEASE PRESSURE after 5 minutes.

VARIATIONS: This method works for most fish filets, although the cook time may need to be increased to accommodate a thicker filet. Salmon, halibut, or tilapia would work very well. Fish tends to have subtle flavor and something as simple as salt and pepper complements it well. However, premixed spice blends make meal prep easy, just check the ingredients for sugar or starchy fillers before purchasing. Excellent all-purpose spice blends, such as Italian, Cajun, Greek, and garlic herb are great. Or, using a tablespoon of your favorite vinaigrette will add some fat as well as flavor.

DAIRY-FREE VARIATION: Replace butter with 1 tablespoon olive oil or avocado oil, plus a little for greasing.

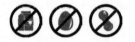

Nutrition Facts	
(amount per serving)	
Energy (calories)	266
Fat	18.1g
Protein	24.4g
Total Carbohydrates	0.1g
Fiber	0g
Net Carbohydrates	0.1g

Macronutrient Breakdown	
Fat	61%
Protein	36%
Carbs	0.1%

CHAPTER 9

Vegetables

Vegetable Broth

Having a base, whether for soups or sauces, that's already got some flavor builds dimension and complexity into a dish. This vegetable stock is perfect when you're looking for something different from the beef or poultry stocks.

MAKES about 3 quarts

2 medium onions, skin-on, halved

2 to 3 large carrots

3 stalks celery

1 tomato, halved

4 to 5 white mushrooms, halved

1 tablespoon (18g) salt

1 tablespoon (9g) whole peppercorns

1 tablespoon (3g) dried thyme

2 teaspoons (2.4g) dried rosemary

1 bay leaf

PREPARE THE POT

1. Add all the ingredients to the pot.

2. Fill the pot three-quarters full with cool water.

3. Close the lid and lock. SEAL the pressure valve.

4. Set to HIGH PRESSURE and cook for 45 minutes.

5. Then NATURAL RELEASE.

6. Pour the stock through a strainer to remove solids.

7. Use immediately or keep in the fridge for a few days. For longer-term storage, store stock in 1-quart Ziploc bags, with the air removed, and keep them in the freezer.

VARIATIONS: Roasting or charring the ingredients beforehand in an oven adds more depth of flavor. Try changing it up and use a leek instead of one of the onions. Garlic and ginger are good for seasoning too, whether used in tandem or individually. In addition to the tomato, add 2 to 3 teaspoons of tomato paste to bring out more umami flavor.

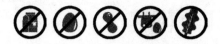

Nutrition facts and macronutrient breakdowns are not included for stocks and broths (see page 26).

Broccoli Cheddar Soup

This broccoli cheddar soup is rich and cheesy—so cheesy it just may convince the pickiest eater to eat broccoli! Enjoy it as a soup or use it as a sauce. Top with a tablespoon of shredded cheddar to mix in at the table.

MAKES 8 (½-cup) servings

3 tablespoons (38g) ghee or salted butter

½ medium onion, chopped

1 clove garlic, minced

1 pound (454g) broccoli florets, plus more to serve

1 teaspoon (6g) salt

½ teaspoon (0.3g) dried sage

2 cups (500mL) chicken stock

½ cup (125mL) heavy cream, 33%

½ cup (125mL) homogenized milk or whole milk

1¼ cups (150g) shredded cheddar cheese, plus more to serve

¼ cup (26g) grated Parmesan cheese

bacon bits, to serve

chopped green onion, to serve

PREPARE THE POT

1. Set the pressure cooker to SAUTÉ.

2. Once hot, melt the ghee or butter.

3. Add the onion and sauté until translucent, about 1½ minutes.

4. Add garlic and sauté until fragrant, about 30 seconds.

5. Add the broccoli, salt, and sage.

6. Stir broccoli every 30 seconds, for about 2 minutes.

7. Pour in the stock and stir to deglaze the pot.

8. Close the lid and lock. SEAL the pressure valve.

9. Set to HIGH PRESSURE and cook for 2 minutes.

10. Then QUICK RELEASE.

11. Add the cream, milk, cheddar cheese, and Parmesan cheese, and stir to combine.

12. Close the lid and lock. SEAL the pressure valve.

13. Set to HIGH PRESSURE and cook for 0 minutes just to bring it up to pressure.

14. Then QUICK RELEASE.

15. Blend the soup in the pot with an immersion blender.

16. Ladle into bowls and serve with bacon bits, more broccoli florets and cheddar cheese, and chopped green onion, if desired.

VARIATIONS: Replace the whole milk with almond or coconut milk to cut the carbs down even more. Add 2 to 4 tablespoons of cream cheese to make this even creamier and cheesier, and to make it even more like a sauce.

VEGETARIAN VARIATION: Make it vegetarian by using vegetable stock instead of chicken stock.

Nutrition Facts	
(amount per serving)	
Energy (calories)	209
Fat	17g
Protein	8.1g
Total Carbohydrates	6.1g
Fiber	1.7g
Net Carbohydrates	4.4g

Macronutrient Breakdown	
Fat	73%
Protein	15%
Carbs	12%

Cauliflower Mash

Cauliflower mash as a keto-friendly substitute for mashed potatoes is a staple at home. It's fast and simple to make. I try to keep this recipe as neutral as possible because it's most often paired with other dishes that are quite flavorful. It's essentially a sauce carrier! And while this mash is great on its own, it's even better with the works: bacon bits, sour cream, chopped green onion, and melted cheddar cheese.

MAKES 8 (½-cup) servings

1 large cauliflower head

¼ cup (56g) butter, preferably salted

¼ cup (60mL) heavy cream, 33%

2 teaspoons (12g) salt

PREPARE THE POT

1. Add 1 cup of water to the pot, and place in the flat wire steamer rack with the handles up.

2. Place the cauliflower head on the rack.

3. Close the lid and lock. SEAL the pressure valve.

4. Set to HIGH PRESSURE and cook for 5 to 6 minutes.

5. Then MANUAL RELEASE PRESSURE after 2 minutes.

6. Carefully remove the cauliflower (it's pretty soft!) by picking up the steamer rack by the handles using mini silicone mitts.

7. Transfer the cauliflower to a bowl.

8. Mash with a potato masher or fork.

9. Carefully drain the excess water, and mix in the butter and cream, and add salt to taste.

VARIATIONS: Instead of using cream, try sour cream or chicken stock. For a flavor boost, add a minced garlic clove or two along with some dried herbs like thyme or dill.

DAIRY-FREE AND VEGAN VARIATION: Use coconut or a flavor-infused olive oil such as a basil or garlic, instead of butter, and use almond or coconut milk instead of heavy cream.

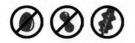

Nutrition Facts	
(amount per serving)	
Energy (calories)	127
Fat	9g
Protein	3.3g
Total Carbohydrates	8.3g
Fiber	3.2g
Net Carbohydrates	5.1g

Macronutrient Breakdown	
Fat	63%
Protein	10%
Carbs	26%

Hickory Alfredo Cauliflower Mash

Cauliflower is such a versatile vegetable and pretty neutral by itself. This cooking method is a little different in that the flavoring, the liquid smoke, is placed in the steaming water. The flavor is subtler than adding the liquid smoke directly to the mash, and the florets pick up the smoky essence like they've been "kissed." The beef stock tames the smoky flavor a little more and gives it a heartier feel. This is a perfect side dish for beef recipes such as the prime rib roast or stews. Top with sour cream and chopped green onions.

MAKES 8 (½-cup) servings

1 large cauliflower head

2 tablespoons (30mL) hickory liquid smoke

½ cup (125mL) beef, chicken, or vegetable stock

⅓ cup (63g) grated Parmesan cheese

¼ cup (62mL) heavy cream, 33%

1 teaspoon (6g) salt

freshly ground pepper

PREPARE THE POT

1. Add 1½ cup water to the pot along with the liquid smoke. Place in the flat wire steamer rack with the handle up.

2. Place the cauliflower head on the rack.

3. Close the lid and lock. SEAL the pressure valve.

4. Set to HIGH PRESSURE and cook for 5 to 6 minutes.

5. Then MANUAL RELEASE PRESSURE after 2 minutes.

6. Carefully remove cauliflower (it's pretty soft!) and transfer to a bowl.

7. Mash with a potato masher or a fork. Drain off any water.

8. Mix in the stock, Parmesan cheese, and heavy cream.

9. Season with salt and pepper to taste.

VARIATION: Use mesquite liquid smoke instead of the hickory, and pair the cauliflower side with a chicken dish.

Nutrition Facts (amount per serving)	
Energy (calories)	94
Fat	5.1g
Protein	5.4g
Total Carbohydrates	6.7g
Fiber	2.5g
Net Carbohydrates	4.2g

Macronutrient Breakdown	
Fat	48.7%
Protein	22.9%
Carbs	28.4%

Cream of Brussels Sprouts Soup with Tarragon, Dill, and Blue Cheese

There are times when I am absolutely amazed by how a pressure cooker infuses flavors, and this soup is a great example. The distinct taste of Brussels sprouts and blue cheese softens and mellows, and brings a unique flavor unto itself.

MAKES 8 (½-cup) servings

2 tablespoons (28g) ghee or salted butter

1 cup (110g) chopped onion (about 1 medium onion)

1 pound (454g) Brussels sprouts, halved

3 cups (750mL) chicken or vegetable stock, divided

1 cup (250mL) cool water

¼ cup (60mL) heavy cream, 33%

2 teaspoons (1.2g) dried tarragon

1 tablespoon (8.9g) fresh dill, plus more to serve

2 teaspoons (12g) salt

½ teaspoon (1.4g) freshly ground pepper

2 tablespoons (27g) crumbled blue cheese

PREPARE THE POT

1. Set the pressure cooker to SAUTÉ.

2. When hot, add the ghee or butter.

3. Once melted, add the onion and a dash of salt. Sauté until softened and translucent, about 1½ minutes.

4. Add the Brussels sprouts, let sit for 30 seconds, then stir. Repeat for 4 minutes or until three-quarters of the sprouts have browned.

5. Pour in 1 cup of the stock and stir to deglaze the pan.

6. Add in the rest of stock along with the water, cream, tarragon, dill, salt, and pepper. Stir well.

7. Cover with the lid and lock. SEAL the pressure valve.

8. Set to HIGH PRESSURE and cook for 12 minutes.

9. Then QUICK RELEASE.

10. Add the blue cheese and stir to combine.

11. Blend with an immersion blender in the pot or transfer to a blender and blend until the soup is a smooth consistency.

12. Serve with a pinch or two of fresh dill.

VARIATIONS: Substitute cabbage or cauliflower for of the Brussels sprouts. Instead of the blue cheese, pick another bold-flavored cheese. Feta is delicious with the Brussels sprouts!

VEGETARIAN VARIATION: Use vegetable stock instead of chicken stock.

VEGAN VARIATION: Using avocado or olive oil instead of ghee or butter. Use vegetable stock in place of chicken stock, and use coconut milk instead of cream. Omit the blue cheese or use a vegan substitute.

Nutrition Facts	
(amount per serving)	
Energy (calories)	100
Fat	6.8g
Protein	3g
Total Carbohydrates	6.9g
Fiber	2.5g
Net Carbohydrates	4.4g

Macronutrient Breakdown	
Fat	60.7%
Protein	2%
Carbs	27%

Cream of Mushroom Soup

Cream of mushroom soup was a childhood favorite of mine, but it came from a can and was mixed with starchy thickening agents. This version is fresh, low-carb, and easily made in the time it takes to open up a can and heat it. It just needs a minute at pressure to let the flavors mingle and soften. Not only a great soup—try serving with a drop of liquid smoke or crumbled bacon on top—but a wonderful ingredient in other recipes too!

MAKES 4 (1-cup) servings

2 tablespoons (28g) ghee, salted butter, or avocado oil

1 medium onion, chopped

12 white or brown mushrooms, sliced

1 teaspoon (6g) salt

½ teaspoon (0.5g) dried thyme

3 cups (750mL) beef, chicken, or vegetable stock, divided

½ teaspoon (2.5mL) Worcestershire sauce

1 cup (250mL) heavy cream, 33%

freshly ground pepper

PREPARE THE POT

1. Set the pressure cooker to SAUTÉ.

2. When hot, add the ghee, butter, or avocado oil.

3. Once melted add the onion and sauté until soft, about 1½ minutes.

4. Add the mushrooms and sauté for 1 minute more.

5. Sprinkle in the salt and thyme, and stir to combine.

6. Pour in ½ cup of the stock and stir to deglaze the pot.

7. Then add the rest of stock and the Worcestershire sauce.

8. Close the lid and lock. SEAL the pressure valve.

9. Set to HIGH PRESSURE and cook for 1 minute.

10. Then MANUAL RELEASE PRESSURE after 1 minute

11. Stir in the cream.

12. Set the pressure cooker to SAUTÉ to warm the soup back up.

13. Cook for about 2 minutes. Stir occasionally to prevent the cream from burning.

14. If desired, break up the mushroom pieces with an immersion blender.

15. Season with salt and pepper to taste.

VARIATION: Instead of using thyme, try oregano. Try different kinds of mushrooms for variety.

VEGAN VARIATION: Make it vegan by using coconut or avocado oil instead of ghee, vegetable stock instead of beef stock, liquid aminos instead of Worcestershire sauce, and coconut milk with cream instead of heavy cream.

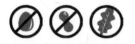

Nutrition Facts	
(amount per serving)	
Energy (calories)	293
Fat	28g
Protein	3.7g
Total Carbohydrates	6.7g
Fiber	1.2g
Net Carbohydrates	5.5g

Macronutrient Breakdown	
Fat	85%
Protein	5%
Carbs	9%

Feta Bacon Brussels Sprouts

My inspiration for this recipe came from many Christmases ago when my aunt brought steamed Brussels sprouts topped with a copious amount of crumbled feta for dinner. The saltiness from the feta seems to balance out the slightest bit of bitterness from the sprouts. My original run had the cook time of 4 minutes, which made the Brussels sprouts a little too soft. I've cut the time in half, but larger sprouts may need an extra minute under pressure. Check for doneness after 2 minutes, and if it needs a little more time, then add a minute under pressure. Add some crumbled bacon on top along with some fresh dill to add another level of flavor.

MAKES 6 (½-cup) servings

2 slices bacon, cut in ½-inch pieces

1 pound (454g) Brussels sprouts, halved

¾ cup (180mL) pork, chicken, or vegetable stock

¼ teaspoon (1.5g) sea salt

6 tablespoons (57g) crumbled feta, or more if desired

PREPARE THE POT

1. Set the pressure cooker to SAUTÉ.

2. Once hot, add the bacon.

3. Stir when it no longer sticks to the pot.

4. Add the Brussels sprouts. Let sit for 30 seconds, then stir. Repeat for about 2 minutes.

5. Pour in the stock, stir to deglaze the pot, and add salt.

6. Cover with the lid and lock. SEAL the pressure valve.

7. Set to HIGH PRESSURE and cook for 2 minutes.

8. Then MANUAL RELEASE PRESSURE after 1 minute.

9. Remove the Brussels sprouts from pot, leaving any liquid behind.

10. Toss with the feta.

11. Place into bowls. Spoon cooking liquid over the top. Serve hot.

VEGETARIAN VARIATION: Make it vegetarian by using ghee instead of bacon, and season to taste before serving.

Nutrition Facts	
(amount per serving)	
Energy (calories)	103
Fat	6g
Protein	5.1g
Total Carbohydrates	7.3g
Fiber	2.9g
Net Carbohydrates	4.4g

Macronutrient Breakdown	
Fat	52%
Protein	20%
Carbs	28%

Palak Paneer (Spinach with Cheese)

I don't use spinach often enough, but when I do, it's so convenient to use the frozen variety. This recipe was a favorite with the taste-testing crew, only they wanted more heat!

MAKES 6 to 7 (¾-cup) servings

Spices

½ teaspoon (1.5g) ground turmeric

1 teaspoon (1.8g) cayenne pepper (add ½ to 1 teaspoon more for more heat)

1 teaspoon (6g) salt

1 teaspoon (3g) garam masala

1 teaspoon (1.8g) ground coriander

⅛ teaspoon (0.5g) ground fenugreek

Palak Paneer

2 tablespoons (25g) ghee, olive oil, or avocado oil

1 medium onion, chopped

2 cloves garlic, minced

2 teaspoons (10g) grated fresh ginger

1 medium tomato, chopped

¼ cup (60mL) coconut milk with cream

2 (10.5oz, 300g) packages frozen spinach

2 cups (400g) cubed paneer cheese

1. Mix the spices together and set aside.

PREPARE THE POT

2. Set the pressure cooker to SAUTÉ.

3. Once hot, add the ghee, olive oil, or avocado oil.

4. Add the onion and sauté until soft and translucent, about 1½ minutes.

5. Add the garlic, ginger, and spice mix.

6. Stir for 1 to 2 minutes to toast and activate the spices.

7. Add the tomato, coconut milk, and frozen spinach.

8. Close the lid and lock. SEAL the pressure valve.

9. Set to HIGH PRESSURE and cook for 10 minutes.

10. Then QUICK RELEASE

11. Break up the spinach with a spoon.

12. If desired, blend with an immersion blender for a smoother texture.

13. Stir in the paneer cheese.

14. Set the pressure cooker to SAUTÉ.

15. Stir for 1 to 2 minutes, until the paneer is warmed through.

VARIATIONS: "Palak" distinctly refers to spinach. To make saag paneer, use other greens such as kale, mustard, or collards in combination with the spinach or without. Add a little nuttiness to the paneer and pan-fry it in a little bit of ghee before adding it to the pressure cooker.

VEGAN VARIATION: Omit the paneer, and use avocado or olive oil instead of ghee.

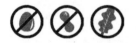

Nutrition Facts	
(amount per serving)	
Energy (calories)	276
Fat	22g
Protein	14g
Total Carbohydrates	6.2g
Fiber	0.9g
Net Carbohydrates	5.3g

Macronutrient Breakdown	
Fat	71%
Protein	20%
Carbs	9%

Pumpkin Coconut Brussels Sprout Soup

With different diets and food sensitivities, cooking for others can be a challenge at times. This recipe was fun to put together and was enjoyed by many. With 4.7g of net carbs, it works in the keto-friendly diet, especially when other macros are in check and you're looking for something a little different.

MAKES 10 (½-cup) servings

Spices

2 teaspoons (2g) dried thyme

½ teaspoon (0.7g) ground cumin

1¾ teaspoons (10.5g) salt

½ teaspoon (1.4g) ground white or black pepper

Soup

2 tablespoons (27g) coconut oil

½ cup (80g) onion, about ½ medium onion, chopped

1 pound (454g) Brussels sprouts, ends cut and cut in half

1 clove garlic, minced

3 cups (750mL) chicken or vegetable stock, divided

½ cup (125mL) coconut milk with cream

1 cup (259g) canned pumpkin puree

salt

1. Mix the spices together and set aside.

PREPARE THE POT

2. Set the pressure cooker to SAUTÉ.

3. When hot, add the coconut oil.

4. Once melted, add the onion and a dash of salt. Sauté until softened, about 1 minute.

5. Add the Brussels sprouts, let sit for 30 seconds, then stir. Repeat for 4 minutes, or until three-quarters of the sprouts have turned bright green or even a little brown.

6. Add the garlic and stir.

7. Pour in 1 cup of stock and stir to deglaze the pot.

8. Stir in the rest of the stock and the coconut milk.

9. Stir in the pumpkin puree.

10. Stir in the spice mix.

11. Close the lid and lock. SEAL the pressure valve.

12. Set to HIGH PRESSURE and cook for 12 minutes.

13. Then QUICK RELEASE.

14. Blend in the pot with an immersion blender, or transfer to a blender and puree until smooth.

15. Season with salt and pepper to taste.

VEGETARIAN AND VEGAN VARIATION: Use vegetable stock instead of chicken stock.

VARIATIONS: To bump up the fat macros a little more, replace the coconut milk with heavy cream. For a little smoky flavor, add some crumbled bacon or a drop of liquid smoke.

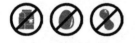

Nutrition Facts	
(amount per serving)	
Energy (calories)	77
Fat	5.4g
Protein	2.2g
Total Carbohydrates	7.3g
Fiber	2.6g
Net Carbohydrates	4.7g

Macronutrient Breakdown	
Fat	56%
Protein	10%
Carbs	33%

Spicy Cauliflower and Zucchini

One of the benefits of pressure cooking is that it takes much less time for flavors to come together that ordinarily would take hours. The challenge is having ingredients that become mushy within minutes of being under pressure. Plus, I can be a little impatient! If you have a lower pressure setting on your pressure cooker, cook this dish for 5 to 7 minutes to give the spices more time to infuse while keeping the veggies just al dente.

MAKES 8 (½-cup) servings

Spices

1 teaspoon (3g) ground turmeric

1 teaspoon (2.3g) paprika

½ teaspoon (1.8g) cayenne pepper

1 teaspoon (6g) salt

½ teaspoon (1.6g) garam masala

½ teaspoon (0.8g) red chile flakes

Cauliflower and Zucchini

2 tablespoons (25g) ghee or butter

½ medium onion, sliced

1 (28oz, 796mL) can diced tomatoes with liquid

1 medium zucchini, cubed (about 3 cups)

½ medium head cauliflower, broken into florets (about 6 cups)

1. Mix the spices together and set aside.

PREPARE THE POT

2. Set the pressure cooker to SAUTÉ.

3. Once hot, add the ghee or butter to melt.

4. Add the onion and sauté until soft, about 1 minute.

5. Add the spice mix and stir for 1 to 2 minutes to heat and activate the spices.

6. Add the tomatoes with their liquid and stir to combine well.

7. Scrape off any bits stuck to the pot and mix them in.

8. Stir in the zucchini and cauliflower.

9. Close the lid and lock. SEAL the pressure valve.

10. Set to HIGH PRESSURE and cook for 1 minute.

11. Then QUICK RELEASE.

12. Top with a spoonful of sauce and serve.

VARIATION: Add more fat! Mix in ½ cup of coconut milk or heavy cream to make a vegetable curry.

DAIRY-FREE AND VEGAN VARIATION: Use coconut oil instead of ghee or butter.

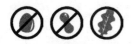

Nutrition Facts	
(amount per serving)	
Energy (calories)	83
Fat	3.8g
Protein	2.8g
Total Carbohydrates	9.2g
Fiber	4g
Net Carbohydrates	5.2g

Macronutrient Breakdown	
Fat	42%
Protein	13%
Carbs	44%

Tomato Soup

I had originally made this soup with heavy cream but wondered whether it would work with coconut milk to make a dairy-free version and brought it to share at work. We were all pleasantly surprised how well it turned out! It's easy and fast to do, especially for many hungry mouths, whether keto or not, to feed. Serve with cheddar cheese sprinkled on top, or with some roasted vegetables, topped with a strong cheese such as feta.

MAKES 6 (1-cup) servings

4 cups (1L) vegetable or chicken stock

1 (28oz, 796mL) can diced tomatoes with liquid

2 teaspoons (12g) salt

½ teaspoon (1.4g) freshly ground pepper

2 teaspoons (4.8g) onion powder

1 cup (250mL) coconut milk with cream

1 tablespoon (16g) tomato paste

2 teaspoons (2g) dried thyme

1 tablespoon (2.1g) dried basil

fresh chopped basil, to serve

cheddar cheese or cheddar cheese crisps, to serve

Parmesan cheese or Parmesan cheese crisps, to serve

PREPARE THE POT

1. Add the stock, tomatoes, salt, pepper, onion powder, coconut milk, tomato paste, thyme, and basil to the pot and stir well to combine.

2. Close the lid and lock. SEAL the pressure valve.

3. Set to HIGH PRESSURE and cook for 5 minutes.

4. Then QUICK RELEASE.

5. Blend in the pot with an immersion blender or transfer to a blender and puree until smooth.

6. Serve topped with fresh basil, and cheddar cheese or cheese crisps or Parmesan cheese or cheese crisps, if desired.

VARIATIONS: Use heavy cream instead of coconut milk for a richer soup and to bump up fats. Add the cream after the cook time, and set the pressure cooker to SAUTÉ for 1 to 2 minutes, stirring to warm up the cream. Then blend with an immersion blender.

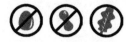

Nutrition Facts	
(amount per serving)	
Energy (calories)	116
Fat	8.1g
Protein	2g
Total Carbohydrates	8.7g
Fiber	0.3g
Net Carbohydrates	8.4g

Macronutrient Breakdown	
Fat	62.7%
Protein	7.1%
Carbs	30.1%

CHAPTER 10
Sweeter Things

Mocha Cheesecake

*Sometimes decadence is required for special occasions or just because!
Finding chocolate chips like Lily's brand, sweetened with stevia and/or with
erythritol helps. There are other great brands out on the market too—just
check the label. I always use Dutch-process cocoa when I can. It's luscious,
rich, and absolutely chocolaty. It can interfere with leaveners in baking, but
it's right at home in this cheesecake. Serve with a little whipped cream and
keto-friendly chocolate chips on top.*

MAKES 12 (1-slice) servings

Crust

1 cup (112g) almond flour

¼ cup (27g) crushed pecans

3 tablespoons (27g) Dutch-process cocoa powder

pinch salt

¼ cup (40g) Swerve sweetener or erythritol

¼ cup (56g) melted butter

Cream Cheese Mixture

2 (8oz, 250g) packages cream cheese, softened and each cut into 8

½ cup (80g) Swerve sweetener or erythritol

1 teaspoon (4g) xylitol

1 cup (200g) stevia- or erythritol-sweetened chocolate chips, melted

Egg Mixture

3 eggs, at room temperature

2 teaspoons (10mL) vanilla extract

¼ cup (60mL) heavy cream, 33%

1 teaspoon (3.3g) dark roast instant coffee or 1 packet Starbucks French Roast Via

⅛ teaspoon (0.8g) salt

PREPARE THE CRUST

1. In a medium bowl, stir together the almond flour, pecans, cocoa, salt, and sweetener.

2. Work in the melted butter. The mixture will be crumbly but will retain its shape when squeezed together.

3. Press mixture evenly into the bottom and a little up the sides of a 6-inch springform pan.

4. Place pan in the freezer while making the filling.

PREPARE THE CREAM CHEESE MIXTURE

5. In a large bowl, cream the cream cheese and both sweeteners with an electric mixer.

6. Slowly add the melted chocolate into the cream cheese mixture while mixing.

7. Once everything is incorporated, set aside.

PREPARE THE EGG MIXTURE

8. In another large bowl, mix with a fork or whisk together the eggs, vanilla, cream, coffee, and salt.

9. On a low mixer setting, slowly pour one-third of the egg mixture into the cream cheese mixture.

10. Scrape down the sides while mixing. Add the remaining egg mixture in two batches, and mix until just smooth.

11. Remove the crust from the freezer and pour in the filling.

12. Cover the top and bottom of the pan with foil.

PREPARE THE POT

13. Add 2 cups of water to the pot. Place in the flat wire steamer rack with the handle up. (Or make a foil sling to put underneath the pan to make it easier to remove.)

14. Carefully set the pan on top of the rack.

15. Close the lid and lock. SEAL the pressure valve.

16. Set to HIGH PRESSURE and cook for 45 minutes.

17. Then MANUAL RELEASE PRESSURE after 10 minutes.

18. Carefully, using handles from steam rack or foil sling, remove the springform pan from the pot.

19. If necessary, wick away any water in the middle of the cake with a paper towel. Check to see if the center is set. It should move like jelly, not like liquid. If not, cook for another 5 minutes.

20. Refrigerate for 2 to 3 hours before removing the cheesecake from the pan. Slice with a knife warmed with hot water.

VARIATIONS: For a chocolate cheesecake, omit the instant coffee. For a chocolate-mint cheesecake, omit the coffee and vanilla extract and add 1 teaspoon peppermint extract. For a chocolate-orange cheesecake, omit the instant coffee and 1 teaspoon of vanilla extract and add 1 teaspoon of orange extract. For a Mexican chocolate cheesecake, omit the instant coffee and 1 teaspoon of vanilla extract, and add 1 tablespoon ground cinnamon, ½ teaspoon cayenne pepper, and ¼ teaspoon ground nutmeg.

Nutrition Facts	
(amount per serving)	
Energy (calories)	357
Fat	32.2g
Protein	7.9g
Total Carbohydrates	11.5g
Fiber	4.2g
Net Carbohydrates	7.3g

Macronutrient Breakdown	
Fat	79%
Protein	8.5%
Carbs	12.5%

Chocolate Peanut Butter Cheesecake

After putting together the Mocha Cheesecake (page 205), I was craving peanut butter, so it was a natural progression to make this recipe. The peanut butter layer uses ricotta cheese instead of cream cheese for a lighter, cakey texture in the middle. My go-to is serving this with whipped cream— you can't go wrong! Or, try something a little different and sprinkle sea salt or, even better, flaked sea salt on top.

MAKES 12 (1-slice) servings

Crust

1 cup (112g) almond flour

¼ cup (27g) crushed pecans

3 tablespoons (27g) Dutch-process cocoa powder

¼ teaspoon (1.5g) sea salt

¼ cup (40g) Swerve sweetener or erythritol

¼ cup (56g) butter, melted

Chocolate Cream Cheese Mixture

½ cup (100g) stevia- or erythritol-sweetened chocolate chips, melted

1 (8oz, 250g) package cream cheese, softened and cut into 8 pieces

¼ cup (40g) Swerve sweetener or erythritol

½ teaspoon (2g) xylitol

Egg Mixture

4 eggs, at room temperature

2 teaspoons (10mL) vanilla extract

¼ cup (60mL) heavy cream, 33%

¼ teaspoon (1.5g) salt

Peanut Butter Ricotta Cheese Mixture

¼ cup (80g) crunchy or smooth natural peanut butter

1½ cups (300g) package ricotta cheese

¼ cup (40g) Swerve sweetener or erythritol

½ teaspoon (2g) xylitol

PREPARE THE CRUST

1. In a medium bowl, stir together the almond flour, pecans, cocoa, salt, and sweetener.

2. Work in the melted butter. The mixture will be crumbly but will retain its shape when squeezed together.

3. Press mixture evenly into the bottom and a little up the sides of a 6-inch springform pan.

4. Place the pan in the freezer while making the filling.

PREPARE THE CHOCOLATE CREAM CHEESE MIXTURE

5. While the melted chocolate is still warm, add the cream cheese to it in a large bowl while stirring to warm the cream cheese.

6. Then add both sweeteners and mix with an electric mixer.

7. Set aside.

PREPARE THE EGG MIXTURE

8. In a large bowl, mix with a fork or whisk together the eggs, vanilla, cream and salt. Divide in half and set aside one half for the peanut butter layer.

9. On a low mixer setting, slowly pour one half of the remaining egg mixture into the chocolate cream cheese mixture. Scrape down the sides while mixing. Add the rest of this portion of the egg mixture.

10. Remove the crust from the freezer and pour half the chocolate batter into the crust. Spread evenly and return to the freezer. Place the other half of chocolate mixture in the fridge.

PREPARE THE PEANUT BUTTER RICOTTA CHEESE MIXTURE

11. With a large spoon or spatula, mix the peanut butter and ricotta cheese together in a large bowl. Then mix in both sweeteners.

12. Add half of reserved egg mixture and stir to incorporate. Add in the rest of the egg mixture, and mix well. Refrigerate for at least 5 minutes.

ASSEMBLE THE REST OF THE CHEESECAKE

13. Remove the crust from freezer, add half of the peanut butter mixture, and carefully spread it evenly over the top of the bottom chocolate layer.

14. Next carefully add in the rest of the chocolate mixture on top of the peanut butter layer, and spread carefully.

15. Cover the top and bottom of the pan with foil.

PREPARE THE POT

16. Add 2 cups of water to the pot. Place in the flat wire steamer rack with the handle up. (Or make a foil sling to put underneath the pan to make it easier to remove.)

17. Carefully set the pan on top of the rack.

18. Close the lid and lock. SEAL the pressure valve.

19. Set to HIGH PRESSURE and cook for 65 minutes.

20. Then MANUAL RELEASE PRESSURE after 5 minutes.

21. Carefully, using handles from the steamer rack or a foil sling, remove the springform pan from the pot.

22. If necessary, wick away any water in the middle of the cake with a paper towel. Check to see if the center is set. It should move like jelly, not like liquid. If not, cook for another 5 minutes.

23. Refrigerate for 4 to 5 hours (overnight is best) before removing the cheesecake from the pan. Slice with a knife warmed with hot water.

Nutrition Facts	
(amount per serving)	
Energy (calories)	343
Fat	29g
Protein	10.6g
Total Carbohydrates	9.6g
Fiber	3.3g
Net Carbohydrates	6.3g

Macronutrient Breakdown	
Fat	76%
Protein	12%
Carbs	11%

New York Cheesecake

A basic New York–style cheesecake is wonderfully indulgent for any recipe repertoire, and you'd never know it's low-carb. A perfect fat bomb to get your good fats in. Great as is or dress it up! Serve with berries or a berry compote and whipped cream. Drizzle with a little bit of sugar-free caramel syrup and sprinkle with sea salt. Or add some whipped cream on top with grated dark chocolate for a little more decadence!

MAKES 12 (1-slice) servings

1 cup (112g) almond flour

¼ cup (27g) crushed pecans

¾ cup (121g) Swerve sweetener or erythritol, divided

¼ cup (56g) butter, melted

2 (8oz, 250g) packages cream cheese, softened

1 teaspoon (4g) xylitol

3 eggs, at room temperature

2 teaspoons (10mL) vanilla extract

¼ cup (60mL) heavy cream, 33%

1. Mix together the almond flour, pecans, and ¼ cup of the Swerve or erythritol.

2. Work in the melted butter. The mixture will be crumbly but will retain its shape when squeezed together.

3. Press the mixture evenly into the bottom and a little up the sides of a 6-inch springform pan.

4. Place pan in the freezer while making the filling.

5. In a large bowl, cream the cream cheese with the remaining ½ cup Swerve or erythritol and the xylitol with an electric mixer. Set aside.

6. In a medium bowl, mix with a fork or whisk together the eggs, vanilla, and cream.

7. On a low mixer setting, slowly pour the egg mixture into the bowl with the cream cheese. Scrape down the sides while mixing. Mix until just smooth.

8. Remove the crust from the freezer and pour the filling into the crust.

9. Cover the top and bottom of the pan with foil.

PREPARE THE POT

10. Add 2 cups of water to the pot. Place in the flat wire steamer rack with the handle up. (Or make a foil sling to put underneath the pan to make it easier to remove.)

11. Carefully set the pan on top of the rack.

12. Close the lid and lock. SEAL the pressure valve.

13. Set to HIGH PRESSURE and cook for 37 minutes.

14. Then MANUAL RELEASE PRESSURE after 10 minutes.

15. Carefully, using the handles from the rack or the foil sling, remove the springform pan from the pot.

16. Check to see if the center is set. It should be solid if jiggled. If not, cook for another 5 minutes.

17. Refrigerate for 2 to 3 hours before removing the cheesecake from the pan. Slice with a knife warmed with hot water.

Nutrition Facts	
(amount per serving)	
Energy (calories)	290
Fat	27.8g
Protein	6.5g
Total Carbohydrates	4.6g
Fiber	1.2g
Net Carbohydrates	3.4g

Macronutrient Breakdown	
Fat	86.3%
Protein	9%
Carbs	4.7%

Pumpkin Spice Cheesecake

This is the third version I made of this cheesecake. My taste-testing crew swore that the two previous versions didn't quite make the cut, but I suspect they just wanted more cheesecake. For an extra-spiced crust, use ¼ teaspoon nutmeg instead of just a pinch. Serve with whipped cream and a little sprinkle of cinnamon and nutmeg on top.

MAKES 12 (1-slice) servings

Spices

1 teaspoon (2.6g) ground cinnamon

¼ teaspoon (0.6g) ground nutmeg

½ teaspoon (0.9g) ground ginger

⅛ teaspoon (0.2g) ground cloves

⅛ teaspoon (0.8g) salt

Crust

1 cup (112g) almond flour

¼ cup (27g) crushed pecans

¼ cup (40g) Swerve sweetener or erythritol

pinch salt

pinch ground nutmeg

¼ cup (56g) butter, melted

Filling

2 (8oz, 250g) packages cream cheese, softened

½ cup (80g) Swerve sweetener or erythritol

1 teaspoon (4g) xylitol

3 eggs, at room temperature

¾ cup (183g) pumpkin puree

2 teaspoons (10mL) vanilla extract

¼ cup (60mL) heavy cream, 33%

1. Mix the spices together and set aside.

PREPARE THE CRUST

2. Mix together the almond flour, pecans, Swerve or erythritol, salt, and nutmeg.

3. Work in the melted butter. The mixture will be crumbly but will retain its shape when squeezed together.

4. Press the mixture evenly into the bottom and a little up the sides of a 6-inch springform pan.

5. Place pan in the freezer while making the filling.

PREPARE THE FILLING

6. In a large bowl, cream the cream cheese with the Swerve or erythritol and the xylitol and spice mix with an electric mixer. Set aside.

7. In a medium bowl, mix with a fork or whisk together the eggs, pumpkin puree, vanilla, and cream.

8. On a low mixer setting, slowly pour the egg mixture into the bowl with the cream cheese. Scrape down the sides while mixing. Mix until just smooth.

9. Remove the crust from the freezer and pour in the filling.

10. Cover the top and bottom of the pan with foil.

PREPARE THE POT

11. Add 2 cups of water to the pot. Place in the flat wire steamer rack with the handle up. (Or make a foil sling to put underneath the pan to make it easier to remove.)

12. Carefully set the pan on top of the rack.

13. Close the lid and lock. SEAL the pressure valve.

14. Set to HIGH PRESSURE and cook for 60 minutes.

15. Then MANUAL RELEASE PRESSURE after 10 minutes.

16. Carefully, using the handles from the rack or the foil sling, remove the springform pan from the pot.

17. Check to see if the center is set. It should be solid if jiggled. If not, cook for another 5 minutes.

18. Refrigerate at least for 2 to 3 hours (overnight is best) before removing cheesecake from pan. Slice with a knife warmed with hot water.

Nutrition Facts	
(amount per serving)	
Energy (calories)	294
Fat	27.1g
Protein	6.4g
Total Carbohydrates	6.1g
Fiber	1.8g
Net Carbohydrates	4.3g

Macronutrient Breakdown	
Fat	83%
Protein	8.7%
Carbs	8.3%

Snickerdoodle Cheesecake Cups

This cheesecake has a more cake-like texture with the addition of ricotta cheese. It's light, a little fluffy but nicely rich. There's no messing around with a crust, although you could add one if you'd like! I keep a few of these in the fridge for when my hubby or I feel like a treat. Serve with some cinnamon sprinkled on top and/or whipped cream.

MAKES 10 (½-cup) servings

1 (8oz, 250g) package cream cheese, softened

½ cup (80g) Swerve sweetener or erythritol

1 teaspoon (4g) xylitol

1½ cups (300g) ricotta cheese

3 eggs, room temperature

¼ cup (60mL) heavy cream, 33%

pinch salt

1 teaspoon (5mL) vanilla extract

1 teaspoon (2.6g) ground cinnamon

PREPARE THE POT

1. Add 2 cups of water to the pot. Place in the flat wire steamer rack with the handle up.

2. In a large bowl, cream the cream cheese with both sweeteners with an electric mixer. Once incorporated, mix in the ricotta cheese. Set aside.

3. In a medium bowl, mix with a fork or whisk together the eggs, cream, salt, vanilla, and cinnamon.

4. On a low mixer setting, slowly pour the egg mixture into the bowl with the cream cheese mixture. Scrape down the sides while mixing. Mix until evenly blended.

5. Pour into ramekins or other half-cup heatproof dishes. Cover the dishes with foil.

6. Position the dishes on the rack. Depending on the dimensions of your dishes, you may be able to stack them. If it is not set, just cook in a couple of batches.

7. Close the lid and lock. SEAL the pressure valve.

8. Set to HIGH PRESSURE and cook for 20 minutes.

9. Then MANUAL RELEASE PRESSURE after 2 minutes.

10. Carefully, using silicon mitts or tongs, remove one ramekin to check if the center is set. It should be solid, if jiggled, and jelly like, not like liquid. If it is not set, cook for another 5 minutes.

11. Refrigerate for 1 to 2 hours before serving.

VARIATION: To make vanilla bean cheesecake cups, omit the cinnamon and add the seeds from one vanilla bean pod.

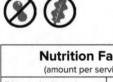

Nutrition Facts	
(amount per serving)	
Energy (calories)	181
Fat	15.5g
Protein	6.9g
Total Carbohydrates	3.5g
Fiber	0.1g
Net Carbohydrates	3.4g

Macronutrient Breakdown	
Fat	76.6%
Protein	15.1%
Carbs	8.3%

Sour Cream Lemon Cheesecake

A refreshing, vibrant cheesecake.

MAKES 12 (1-slice) servings

Crust

1 cup (112g) almond flour

¼ cup (27g) crushed pecans

¼ cup (40g) Swerve sweetener or erythritol

¼ cup (56g) melted butter

Filling

2 (8oz, 250g) packages cream cheese, softened each cut into 8

¾ cup (121g) Swerve sweetener or erythritol

1 teaspoon (4g) xylitol

2 eggs, at room temperature

1 teaspoon (5mL) vanilla extract

2½ tablespoons (37.5mL) lemon juice

2 teaspoons (4g) lemon zest (from about 2 lemons)

Topping

1 cup (250g) sour cream

¼ cup (40g) Swerve sweetener or erythritol

1 teaspoon (2g) lemon zest

1 teaspoon (5mL) vanilla extract

PREPARE THE CRUST

1. In a medium bowl, mix together the almond flour, pecans, and Swerve or erythritol.

2. Work in the melted butter. The mixture will be crumbly but will retain its shape when squeezed together.

3. Press the mixture evenly into the bottom and a little up the sides of a 6-inch springform pan.

4. Place pan in the freezer while making the filling.

PREPARE THE FILLING

5. In a large bowl, cream the cream cheese with the Swerve or erythritol and the xylitol with an electric mixer. Set aside.

6. In a medium bowl, mix with a fork or whisk together the eggs, vanilla, and lemon juice and zest.

7. On a low mixer setting, slowly pour the egg mixture into the bowl with the cream cheese mixture. Scrape down the sides while mixing. Mix until just smooth.

8. Remove the crust from freezer and pour in the filling.

9. Cover the top and bottom of the pan with foil.

PREPARE THE POT

10. Add 1½ cups of water to the pot. Place in the flat wire steamer rack with the handle up. (Or make a foil sling to put underneath the pan to make it easier to remove.)

11. Carefully set the pan on top of the rack.

12. Close the lid and lock. SEAL the pressure valve.

13. Set to HIGH PRESSURE and cook for 60 minutes.

14. Then MANUAL RELEASE PRESSURE after 2 minutes.

15. Carefully, using the handles from the rack or the foil sling, remove the springform pan from the pot.

16. Check to see if the center is set. It should be solid if jiggled. If not, cook for another 5 minutes.

17. Refrigerate for 2 to 3 hours.

PREPARE THE TOPPING

18. Mix together the sour cream, Swerve or erythritol, lemon zest, and vanilla.

19. Refrigerate until ready to serve cheesecake.

20. Run a hot knife along the sides of the pan. Remove the ring.

21. Pour half of the topping over the top of the cheesecake.

22. Slice into 12 with a hot knife.

23. Serve with an extra dollop of topping.

VARIATION: Try replacing the lemon juice and zest with lime.

Nutrition Facts (amount per serving)	
Energy (calories)	296
Fat	28.7g
Protein	6.1g
Total Carbohydrates	5.1g
Fiber	1.2g
Net Carbohydrates	3.9g

Macronutrient Breakdown	
Fat	85%
Protein	8%
Carbs	6.7%

Coconut Custard

I was originally going to use heavy cream for this recipe to make just a basic vanilla custard, but I ran out of cream and had a few cans of coconut milk with cream lying around. I was really happy with the way it turned out. It's a little lighter than a regular custard, and coconut is just so yummy. It was serendipitous! Serve with berries and/or whipped cream or whipped coconut cream.

MAKES 4 (½-cup) servings

1 (13½oz, 400mL) can coconut milk with cream

3 whole eggs, at room temperature

1 egg yolk, at room temperature

1 teaspoon (5mL) vanilla extract

⅓ cup (52g) Swerve sweetener or erythritol

1 teaspoon (4g) xylitol

pinch salt

PREPARE THE POT

1. Add 2 cups of water to the pot. Place in the flat wire steamer rack with the handle up.

2. In a bowl, blend with an electric mixer the coconut milk with its cream to break up the large chunks.

3. Once blended, add the whole eggs, egg yolk, vanilla, both sweeteners, and salt, and blend until mixed.

4. Pour into half-cup ramekins. Cover with foil.

5. Carefully position the ramekins on the rack in the pressure cooker.

6. Close the lid and lock. SEAL the pressure valve.

7. Set to HIGH PRESSURE and cook for 18 minutes.

8. Then MANUAL RELEASE PRESSURE after 1 to 2 minutes.

9. With tongs, remove the ramekins and refrigerate for 2 to 3 hours until set.

VARIATIONS: Use heavy whipping cream along with unsweetened almond or cashew milk to cut down the fat a little. And there's nothing like the flavor of vanilla bean! Split a 2-inch (5 cm) piece of vanilla bean pod and scrape out the seeds. Use it instead of the extract.

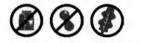

Nutrition Facts (amount per serving)	
Energy (calories)	257
Fat	24.3g
Protein	6.5g
Total Carbohydrates	3.2g
Fiber	0g
Net Carbohydrates	3.2g

Macronutrient Breakdown	
Fat	85%
Protein	10%
Carbs	5%

Coconut Lime Custard

Most often with coconut milk, the cream separates. It was a little challenging to blend it in with the milk to get it nice and uniform. But that may not be a bad thing! The taste-testing crew enjoyed the little bits of coconut cream in the custard, but you can decide your preference. Top with whipped coconut cream and/or coconut flakes.

MAKES 4 (½-cup) servings

1 (13½oz, 400mL) can coconut milk with cream

3 eggs, at room temperature

1 teaspoon (5mL) vanilla extract

⅓ cup (95g) Swerve sweetener or erythritol

1 teaspoon (5g) Xylitol

4 tablespoons (70mL) lime juice

pinch salt

PREPARE THE POT

1. Add 2 cups of water to the pot. Place in the flat wire steamer rack with the handle up.

2. In a bowl, blend with an electric mixer the coconut milk with its cream to break up the large chunks.

3. Once blended, add the eggs, vanilla, both sweeteners, lime juice, and salt, and blend until mixed.

4. Pour into half-cup ramekins.

5. Cover with foil.

6. Carefully position the ramekins on the rack in the pressure cooker.

7. Close and the lid and lock. SEAL the pressure valve.

8. Set to HIGH PRESSURE and cook for 18 minutes.

9. Then MANUAL RELEASE PRESSURE after 1 to 2 minutes.

10. With tongs, remove the ramekins and refrigerate for 2 to 3 hours until set.

VARIATIONS: Use other citrus fruits lower on the carb scale, such as key limes and lemons. Add in some toasted coconut in with the custard for added texture. Or make mini coconut lime pies! Put in an almond or mixed nut crust, then the custard. After refrigeration, top with some whipped coconut cream and coconut flakes. To bump it up even more on the decadence scale, use a kitchen torch (or creme brulée torch) to toast the coconut before serving.

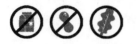

Nutrition Facts	
(amount per serving)	
Energy (calories)	242
Fat	23.5g
Protein	6.1g
Total Carbohydrates	4.6g
Fiber	0.1g
Net Carbohydrates	4.5g

Macronutrient Breakdown	
Fat	83%
Protein	9%
Carbs	7%

Dark Chocolate Brownies

Making these brownies was fun! Since they were made in nine separate ramekins, I cooked them all for different times then brought them to the taste-testing crew. I didn't find one perfect cook time because everyone preferred something a little different. Cook for 35 minutes for a more cakey brownie. Go for 28 minutes for something fudgy. It's up to you! This is quite the fat bomb, with a cup of butter. The butter rises to the top while cooking and resettles in upon cooling, about 15 minutes. It's what gives these the brownies their fudgy consistency. Top with a little whipped cream and chopped nuts to serve.

MAKES 9 (½-cup) servings

1 cup (224g) melted butter

1 tablespoon (15mL) vanilla extract

3 eggs, at room temperature

1 cup (162g) Swerve sweetener or erythritol

1 teaspoon (4g) xylitol

pinch salt

1⅓ cups (150g) almond flour

¾ cup (64g) Dutch-process cocoa powder, sifted

¼ cup (27g) crushed pecans

1. In a large bowl, mix together the butter, vanilla, and eggs.

2. Whisk in both sweeteners and the salt.

3. In a medium bowl, whisk together the almond flour and cocoa.

4. Slowly, while whisking, gradually add the dry ingredients to the wet. As the mixture becomes thicker, change to a spatula or spoon to make it easier to mix.

5. Stir in the pecans.

6. Pour into half-cup ramekins or any small heatproof containers. Cover containers with foil.

PREPARE THE POT

7. Add 2 cups of water to the pot. Place in the flat wire steamer rack with the handle up.

8. Carefully set the ramekins on top of the rack. You may be able to stagger and stack them, depending on the size of your dishes.

9. Close the lid and lock. SEAL the pressure valve.

10. Set to HIGH PRESSURE and cook for 35 minutes. (If you want it more fudgy, cook for 28 minutes, and to make it more molten, cook for just 20 minutes!)

11. Then MANUAL RELEASE PRESSURE after 2 minutes.

12. Carefully, using tongs or mini silicone mitts, remove the ramekins from the pot.

13. Let sit for 15 to 30 minutes at room temperature for the butter to reincorporate.

VARIATIONS: Instead of pecans, try walnuts, hazelnuts, macadamias, or pumpkin seeds.

NUT-FREE VARIATION: Omit the nuts and replace them with chocolate chips.

Nutrition Facts	
(amount per serving)	
Energy (calories)	358
Fat	33g
Protein	7.3g
Total Carbohydrates	8.1g
Fiber	4.1g
Net Carbohydrates	4g

Macronutrient Breakdown	
Fat	82%
Protein	8%
Carbs	9%

Blondies

I wonder if the concept of the "blondie" came about when someone wanted to make brownies but ran out of cocoa powder! No matter their origin, it's a nice twist to have something that's like a brownie but isn't quite. As with the dark chocolate brownies, after the cook time, the butter rises to the surface. Just let stand for a few minutes for the butter to reincorporate. You may want to try a shorter cook time here if you want a fudgier consistency. To serve, melt some low-carb-friendly chocolate chips and drizzle chocolate over the top.

MAKES 9 (½-cup) servings

¾ cup (170g) melted butter

3 eggs, at room temperature

1 teaspoon (5mL) vanilla extract

1 tablespoon (15mL) maple extract

1 cup (162g) Swerve sweetener or erythritol

1 teaspoon (4g) xylitol

pinch salt

1⅓ cups (150g) almond flour

¼ cup (27g) crushed pecans

1. In a large bowl, mix together the butter and eggs.

2. Whisk in the vanilla and maple extracts, then whisk in both sweeteners and the salt.

3. Mix in almond flour, then stir in the pecans.

4. Pour into half-cup ramekins or any small heat-proof containers.

5. Tap the containers on the countertop to help the mixture to settle.

6. Cover the containers with foil.

PREPARE THE POT

7. Add 2 cups of water to the pot. Place in the flat wire steamer rack with the handle up.

8. Carefully set the ramekins on the rack. You may be able to stagger and stack them depending on the size of your dishes.

9. Close the lid and lock. SEAL the pressure valve.

10. Set to HIGH PRESSURE and cook for 35 minutes.

11. Then MANUAL RELEASE PRESSURE after 2 minutes.

12. Carefully, using tongs or mini silicone mitts, remove the ramekins from pot.

13. Let sit for 15 to 30 minutes at room temperature for the butter to reincorporate.

VARIATION: Try changing up the nut flours by using hazelnut flour alone or mixing it with the almond flour.

Nutrition Facts	
(amount per serving)	
Energy (calories)	279
Fat	27.2g
Protein	6g
Total Carbohydrates	3.9g
Fiber	2g
Net Carbohydrates	1.9g

Macronutrient Breakdown	
Fat	88%
Protein	6%
Carbs	3.9%

Mexican Chocolate Pots de Crème

This is a perfect treat for when you're looking for something at the end of the day and have room for some fats, a few more net carbs, and of course, some chocolate. Try serving with a little whipped cream and a mix of cocoa and cinnamon sprinkled on top.

MAKES 9 (½-cup) servings

3 cups (750mL) heavy cream, 33%

6 egg yolks

½ cup (80g) Swerve sweetener or erythritol

1 teaspoon (4g) xylitol

⅛ teaspoon (0.7g) salt

1 teaspoon (5mL) vanilla extract

¾ cup (150g) stevia- or erythritol-sweetened chocolate chips

4 teaspoon (11.4g) ground cinnamon

¼ teaspoon (0.4g) cayenne pepper

⅛ teaspoon (0.2g) ground nutmeg

1. In a large bowl, whisk together the cream, egg yolks, both sweeteners, salt, and vanilla. Set aside.

2. In another large bowl with the melted chocolate, whisk in the cinnamon, cayenne, and nutmeg.

3. While whisking the chocolate, slowly add the cream mixture.

4. After all the cream has been incorporated, pour into half-cup size ramekins or any small heatproof containers. Cover containers with foil.

PREPARE THE POT

5. Add 2 cups of water to the pot. Place in the flat wire steamer rack with the handle up.

6. Carefully set the ramekins on top of the rack. You may be able to stagger and stack them, depending on the size of your dishes.

7. Close the lid and lock. SEAL the pressure valve.

8. Set to HIGH PRESSURE and cook for 15 minutes.

9. Then MANUAL RELEASE PRESSURE after 10 minutes.

10. Carefully, using tongs or mini silicone mitts, remove the ramekins from the pot.

11. Refrigerate for 2 to 3 hours.

VARIATIONS: For chocolate pots de crème, leave out the cinnamon, nutmeg, and cayenne. For chocolate chile pots de crème, leave out the cinnamon and nutmeg, and add ½ teaspoon or more of cayenne pepper.

Nutrition Facts	
(amount per serving)	
Energy (calories)	398
Fat	38g
Protein	4g
Total Carbohydrates	9.4g
Fiber	2.8g
Net Carbohydrates	6.5g

Macronutrient Breakdown	
Fat	86%
Protein	4%
Carbs	9%

Personal Protein Cheesecakes

The idea for this recipe came to me when my husband was looking for something sweet but also wanted some protein. I'm also seeing more and more ketogenic-fueled athletes out there who are looking for more keto-friendly foods to fuel their bodies. What's great about using protein isolates is that they've been purified and for the most part contain only protein. The carb content is really low, if not negligible for some. Just be sure to read the label. You may want to try these cheesecakes with a flavored isolate protein powder, but I suggest doing a small test batch to see if the flavors hold up in the heat. Serve with a little whipped cream.

MAKES 5 (½-cup) servings

½ cup (80g) Swerve sweetener or erythritol

1 (8oz, 250g) package cream cheese, softened and each cut into 8

2 scoops (72g) isolate protein powder

1 teaspoon (5mL) vanilla extract

2 eggs

¼ cup (60mL) heavy cream, 33%

1. Use an electric mixer to cream the sweetener with the cream cheese and protein powder in a large bowl.

2. In a medium bowl, mix together the vanilla, eggs, and cream.

3. Slowly add the egg mixture to the cream cheese, mixing until all the egg mixture is incorporated.

4. Pour into half-cup ramekins and cover with foil.

PREPARE THE POT

5. Add 2 cups of water to the pot. Place in the flat wire steam rack with the handle up.

6. Carefully position the ramekins on the rack in the pressure cooker.

7. Close the lid and lock. SEAL the pressure valve.

8. Set to HIGH PRESSURE and cook for 20 minutes.

9. Then MANUAL RELEASE PRESSURE after 1 to 2 minutes.

10. With tongs, remove the ramekins and refrigerate for 2 to 3 hours until set. Or leave them overnight in the fridge as they become more like cake as they sit.

VARIATIONS: With so many different flavors and kinds of protein powders available, you can experiment using different flavor combinations, such as chocolate mint, chocolate mocha, Creamsicle, etc. The possibilities are endless.

Nutrition Facts (amount per serving)	
Energy (calories)	298
Fat	24g
Protein	17.5g
Total Carbohydrates	3.5g
Fiber	1.8g
Net Carbohydrates	1.7g

Macronutrient Breakdown	
Fat	72%
Protein	23%
Carbs	4.6%

Vanilla Bean Panna Cotta

This panna cotta is wonderfully luscious and quite the no-guilt treat! All the panna cotta recipes in this book call for egg whites from a carton. The egg whites from the carton are more liquidy, as they've been broken up a bit and strained, unlike the whites straight from an egg. I strongly recommend picking up the carton. Using 4 egg whites (½ cup) gives a nice firm texture to the panna cotta. I've also used 2 egg whites (¼ cup) and the texture is more like a pudding consistency. It's different, but also good! To serve, you can't go wrong with whipped cream and a few dark chocolate curls.

MAKE 4 (½-cup) servings

¾ cup (185mL) heavy cream, 33%

⅓ cup (80mL) unsweetened almond milk

2-inch piece vanilla bean pod with seeds scraped

2 tablespoons (24g) Swerve sweetener or erythritol

4 egg whites (½ cup, 126g), preferably from a carton

PREPARE THE POT

1. Add 2 cups of water to the pot. Place in the flat wire steamer rack with the handle up.

2. Place the heavy cream, almond milk, vanilla bean seeds, vanilla bean pod, and sweetener into a saucepan and gently warm on the stove over medium-low heat while stirring. Once the initial signs of steam appear, remove from the heat. Remove and discard the vanilla bean pod.

3. Take 2 or 3 tablespoons of cream mixture and stir it into the egg whites to warm them up a little.

4. Then slowly, while stirring, add the rest of the cream mixture.

5. Pour into 4 half-cup ramekins. Cover with foil.

6. Carefully position the ramekins on the rack in the pressure cooker.

7. Close the lid and lock. SEAL the pressure valve.

8. Set to HIGH PRESSURE and cook for 7 minutes.

9. Then MANUAL RELEASE PRESSURE after 4 to 5 minutes.

10. With tongs, remove the ramekins and refrigerate for 2 to 3 hours until set.

Nutrition Facts	
(amount per serving)	
Energy (calories)	171
Fat	16.6g
Protein	3.9g
Total Carbohydrates	1.7g
Fiber	0.2g
Net Carbohydrates	1.5g

Macronutrient Breakdown	
Fat	87%
Protein	9%
Carbs	4%

Green Tea Panna Cotta

One thing I miss being on the keto diet is green tea ice cream. After making Vanilla Bean Panna Cotta (page 234), I thought to try adding matcha powder. It worked pretty well and just about does the trick for my craving! For a stronger green tea flavor, add ½ to 1 teaspoon more matcha powder. Serve with whipped cream and a sprinkle of matcha powder on top.

MAKES 4 (½-cup) servings

¾ cup (185mL) heavy cream, 33%

⅓ cup (80mL) unsweetened almond milk

½ teaspoon (2.5mL) vanilla extract

2 tablespoons (30g) Swerve sweetener or erythritol

1 teaspoon (2g) matcha green tea powder

4 egg whites (½ cup, 126g), preferably from a carton

PREPARE THE POT

1. Add 2 cups of water to the pot. Place in the flat wire steamer rack with the handle up.

2. Place the cream, almond milk, vanilla, and sweetener in a saucepan and gently warm over the stove on medium-low heat, stirring. Once the initial signs of steam appear, remove from the heat.

3. Place the matcha into a small bowl or large mug. Add 2 ounces (60mL) of the warm cream to the bowl and whisk until all the lumps are gone and it becomes like a paste.

4. Add the matcha paste to the rest of the warmed cream and stir well.

5. Stir 2 or 3 tablespoons of cream mix into the egg whites and to warm them up a little. Then slowly, while stirring, add the rest of the cream mixture.

6. Pour into 4 half-cup ramekins. Cover with foil.

7. Carefully position the ramekins on rack in the pressure cooker.

8. Close the lid and lock. SEAL the pressure valve.

9. Set to HIGH PRESSURE and cook for 7 minutes.

10. Then MANUAL RELEASE PRESSURE after 4 to 5 minutes.

11. With tongs, remove the ramekins and refrigerate for 2 to 3 hours until set.

Nutrition Facts	
(amount per serving)	
Energy (calories)	172
Fat	16.6g
Protein	3.9g
Total Carbohydrates	1.6g
Fiber	0.2g
Net Carbohydrates	1.4g

Macronutrient Breakdown	
Fat	87%
Protein	9%
Carbs	4%

Lemon Panna Cotta

Using lemon extract and real lemon zest will get the zing in this panna cotta without the cream curdling. If you want more lemon flavor, add a little more zest. Serve with fresh whipped cream and fresh lemon zest.

MAKES 4 (½-cup) servings

¾ cup (185mL) heavy cream, 33%

⅓ cup (80mL) unsweetened almond milk

1 teaspoon (5mL) vanilla extract

1½ teaspoons (6.3g) lemon extract

2 tablespoons (24g) Swerve sweetener or erythritol

4 egg whites (½ cup, 126g), preferably from a carton

¼ teaspoon (0.5g) lemon zest

PREPARE THE POT

1. Add 2 cups of water to the pot. Place in the flat wire steamer rack with the handle up.

2. Place the heavy cream, almond milk, vanilla, and lemon extract along with the sweetener in a saucepan and gently warm over medium-low heat on the stove while stirring. Once the initial signs of steam appear, remove from the heat.

3. Take 2 or 3 tablespoons of cream mixture and stir into the egg whites to warm them up. Then slowly, while stirring, add the rest of the cream mix.

4. Stir in the lemon zest.

5. Pour into 4 half-cup ramekins. Cover with foil.

6. Carefully position the ramekins on the rack in the pressure cooker.

7. Close the lid and lock. SEAL the pressure valve.

8. Set to HIGH PRESSURE and cook for 7 minutes.

9. Then MANUAL RELEASE PRESSURE after 4 to 5 minutes.

10. With tongs, remove ramekins and refrigerate for 2 to 3 hours until set.

VARIATION: Use orange extract and orange zest for a Creamsicle flavor.

Nutrition Facts	
(amount per serving)	
Energy (calories)	172
Fat	16.6g
Protein	3.9g
Total Carbohydrates	1.8g
Fiber	0.3g
Net Carbohydrates	1.5g

Macronutrient Breakdown	
Fat	87%
Protein	9%
Carbs	4%

London Fog Panna Cotta

I'm big fan of London fog lattes, which is Earl Grey tea with steamed milk and vanilla syrup, but I haven't had one since switching to the keto diet. Thinking of panna cotta flavors, this was a natural choice. With the Earl Grey tea I used, there were a few little tea bits left in the cream after straining. I didn't mind it, but you may want to strain it more than once. Serve with whipped cream and/or fresh berries.

MAKES 4 (½-cup) servings

¾ cup (185mL) heavy cream, 33%

⅓ cup (80mL) unsweetened almond milk

Earl Grey tea leaves from 1 tea bag

1 teaspoon (5mL) vanilla extract

2 tablespoons (24g) Swerve sweetener or erythritol

4 egg whites (½ cup, 126g), preferably from a carton

pinch salt

PREPARE THE POT

1. Add 2 cups of water to the pot. Place in the flat wire steamer rack with the handle up.

2. Place the heavy cream, almond milk, and Earl Grey tea leaves into a saucepan and gently warm over medium-low heat on the stove while stirring. Once the initial signs of steam appear, remove from the heat.

3. Strain through a couple of layers of cheesecloth and discard the tea.

4. Stir the vanilla, sweetener, and salt into the cream mixture until dissolved. (Reheat slightly if needed.)

5. Take 2 or 3 tablespoons of the cream mixture and stir into the egg whites to warm them up a little.

6. Then slowly, while stirring, add the rest of the cream mixture.

7. Pour into 4 half-cup ramekins. Cover with foil.

8. Carefully position the ramekins on the rack in the pressure cooker.

9. Close the lid and lock. SEAL the pressure valve.

10. Set to HIGH PRESSURE and cook for 7 minutes.

11. Then MANUAL RELEASE PRESSURE after 4 to 5 minutes.

12. With tongs, remove the ramekins and refrigerate for 2 to 3 hours.

VARIATIONS: Try other black teas but without citrus, as it may curdle. You can also try varying the texture by using fewer egg whites. Using two gives a consistency more like a thick pudding than a panna cotta.

Nutrition Facts	
(amount per serving)	
Energy (calories)	171
Fat	16.6g
Protein	3.9g
Total Carbohydrates	1.7g
Fiber	0.2g
Net Carbohydrates	1.5g

Macronutrient Breakdown	
Fat	87%
Protein	9%
Carbs	4%

Acknowledgments

This book wouldn't be possible without the help of many people.

First is Ulysses Press for offering me the opportunity to write my first book. Thank you to everyone who helped put it all together. I'm in awe of what you do and am humbled that you chose me.

Second is my friend Shaela, without whose experience and wisdom I wouldn't have accepted this opportunity with the confidence and knowledge of the amazing experience ahead of me.

Third is my taste-testing crew at work—without all you guys (you know who you are!) I would need to buy an additional freezer! Thank you for letting me cook for you and for all your feedback and suggestions, and even testing some recipes. There just might be a Keto Pumpkin Spice Cheesecake V4.0 in your future!

Fourth are my friends and family who have supported and encouraged me through taste-testing recipes and offering advice but also by just being there when I needed an ear.

A big shout-out to the *Thriving on Low Carb* blog, Facebook, Twitter, and Instagram fans, all of whom I have teased with pictures of my recipe trials and successes. It's here!

Finally is my dear husband, Jeffrey, who has tasted almost every single recipe and supported me through the kitchen chaos. He has been patient through my very late keto cheesecake–making nights with both Instant Pots going at full capacity.

Special mention goes to the Edwards Crossing Starbucks crew, who have kept me going with caffeine and tea while slogging through endless nutritional information and calculations for weeks. And also to Marble Hill Potters for graciously loaning me beautiful pieces of pottery on which to photograph my food.

About the Author

Aileen Ablog discovered the ketogenic diet when she was faced with a future of health ailments. She needed to lose weight and change her eating habits. Within a few months of weight loss and increased energy, she realized this was more than just a diet; it became a lifestyle.

A science geek at heart, Aileen created the blog *Thriving on Low Carb* (thrivingonlowcarb.com) initially to document her journey, but it has since become a resource to help others use the ketogenic diet to make positive health changes.

She lives in Chilliwack, BC, with her husband, Jeffrey, and sassy cat, Lucy. By day she works at the University of the Fraser Valley as a chemistry lab technician. She enjoys cooking, watching movies, and more recently, weight lifting. Rumor has it that Aileen takes her Instant Pot everywhere she goes!